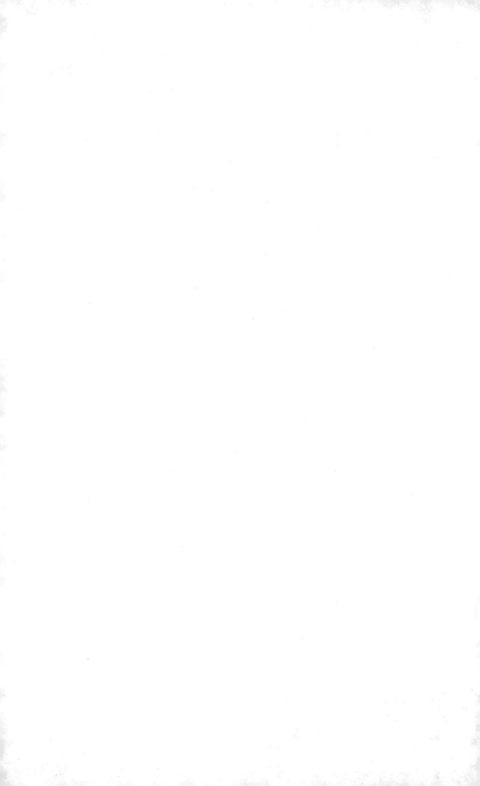

SPORTSWISE:

An Essential Guide for Young Athletes, Parents, and Coaches

SPORTSWISE:

An Essential Guide for Young Athletes, Parents, and Coaches

— ●●● —

Lyle J. Micheli, M.D.,
with Mark D. Jenkins

Houghton Mifflin Company
Boston · 1990

For information about permission to reproduce selections from
this book, write to Permissions, Houghton Mifflin Company,
2 Park Street, Boston, Massachusetts 02108.

Library of Congress Cataloging-in-Publication Data

Micheli, Lyle J.
Sportswise: an essential guide for young athletes, parents, and
coaches / Lyle J. Micheli with Mark D. Jenkins.
p.   cm.
ISBN 0-395-51608-0
ISBN 0-395-56408-5 (pbk.)
1. Sports for children.   2. Sports for children—Accidents and
injuries—Prevention.   √3. Sports for children—Safety measures.
4. Pediatric sports medicine.   I. Jenkins, Mark D.   II. Title.
III. Title: Sportswise: an essential guide for young athletes,
parents, and coaches.
GV709.2.M53   1990   90-34257
796'.01922—dc20   CIP

Printed in the United States of America

BP 10 9 8 7 6 5 4 3 2 1

I have used a number of cases from my practice to illustrate and
emphasize particular points about preventing injuries to our sports-
active children. I have altered all names and, in some cases, family
characteristics to ensure the privacy of these young athletes, who
have taught me so much.

The poem on page 222 is reprinted from *The Reins of Life* by John
Anthony Davis (J. A. Allen & Co., 1 Lower Grosvenor Place, Lon-
don SW1W OEL).

To my daughters Amanda and Lisa, who have helped me gain a special understanding of the sports-active child

Contents

Preface

One of the most difficult balancing acts we face as parents is to try to make sure that our children have safe and successful sports experiences. If we make sports too "safe" we may be robbing our youngsters of physical and emotional challenges they need to become happy, healthy adults. But if we push them too hard to achieve "success" in sports we may cause them physical and psychological injury. This dilemma captures the essence of parenthood: allowing our children to mature while at the same time looking out for their safety.

Although a recent study revealed that over 90 percent of parents want their children to participate in sports, many parents express concern about the potential for physical and psychological harm in organized sports programs. In over twenty years of treating young athletes I've met thousands of distraught parents who have been inundated with horror stories about the dangers in children's sports. Many of them bring me newspaper clippings describing the latest calamity: "Twelve-Year-Old Football Star Sustains Career-Ending Knee Injury," "Teen Quits Tennis Due to Burn-Out," and the perennial "Brawl Erupts among Rival Little League Parents." I've seen or heard them all!

So before we go any further, you should know where I stand.

I'm a passionate advocate of youth sports. You might find that surprising, given that I've spent the better part of my life treating youngsters with serious sports injuries. But you've heard the expression "Good news doesn't sell," haven't you? It applies to children's sports. All the calamitous headlines and "new wives' tales" obscure the fact that millions of kids derive immense pleasure from sports. At this moment countless boys and girls are impatiently tugging on their uniforms to go out and have fun with their friends in an environment where getting hot and dirty and having fun is just as important as hitting a home run or shooting a goal. I'm a firm believer in the benefits of sports for children. Children love to be active — any parent who's dressed up their kids for a special occasion and then tried to keep them clean and quiet knows this. Your youngster's body is saying go, go, go in its growing stages because it needs physical activity to stimulate proper growth. Kids also love to compete. You don't need an adult in charge with a whistle and a bullhorn to get children to start a fiercely competitive game. Put ten children in a field with a bat and ball or even nothing at all and in ten minutes a game will be going on. You may not recognize that game, but it will probably have teams, rules, and scoring.

My own childhood was filled with sports, setting the stage for four wonderful years playing football, lacrosse, rugby, and boxing at Harvard. I still find time to dust off my cleats for an occasional game of "veterans' rugby." Both my daughters are enthusiastic athletes and dancers, and I've been behind them every hop, step, and pirouette of the way! If I weren't such a staunch supporter of sports I wouldn't have made the prevention and treatment of sports injuries my life's work.

But I'm not so gung ho that I can't recognize the profound changes taking place in children's sports and the problems some of these changes are creating. Children's sports today are much different from the games we and our parents played in childhood. Unlike the free play and sandlot sports that once dominated the spare time of American children, now an astonishing 30 million of this country's 45 million youth participate in non-school *organized* sports. The scope of children's sports has widened dramatically. No longer are kids confined to traditional team sports like football, basketball, and baseball; now we see high school distance runners, bikers, and cross-country skiers. One of the most profound changes we've seen has been the massive expansion in sports opportunities for girls and women. Not only are there more opportunities for both boys and girls, but the competition is far more intense. Once children competed for the sake of competition; now there are trophies — big trophies — to be won. I've actually heard talk recently of a Baby Olympics.

One of the undesirable side effects of the explosion in organized competitive sports for children has been a dramatic rise in the incidence and range of sports injuries. Talk of shin splints, stress fractures, and tendinitis was once confined to the pro athletes' locker room; now it can be heard in the high school classroom.

I spend at least four days a week in surgery. Many of the operations I perform are to correct sports injuries. Although developing new surgical techniques is stimulating, challenging, and valuable work, there is also a great need for *preventive* sports medicine. For sports-active children — and their parents — preventing injuries is certainly better than curing them. The alternative, after all, represents pain, inconvenience, and expense! And injuries can have serious long-term consequences for a child's growth. Modern sports medicine tries to prevent these injuries from happening in the first place. Parents should become part of this prevention process.

In this book I discuss the key question "What is fitness?" I also define and explain a number of concepts such as risk factors and the overload principle. Two themes that you will hear throughout the book are that there's been an explosion in children's sports and at the same time that American children are more unfit than ever before. How can both these statements be true? I'll explain why they are, and why injuries are the inevitable consequence of unfit children participating in these new, intense programs.

It's precisely because I believe in the benefits of sports for life that I'm concerned about intense sports programs for children and their potential for physical and psychological harm. A successful sports experience establishes an interest in sports and health fitness activities for life. Unfortunately, too many children drop out of sports because of injury or competitive stress or are forced out because a program is overly elitist. Many of these dropouts are lost to sports forever and end up leading extremely sedentary lives, with all the disastrous health consequences that follow.

The good news is that we can change the way many of these sports programs are run by educating ourselves about sports, preventive sports medicine, and the sports psychology of child athletes. With this knowledge, parents can make sports both healthy and wholesome for their children.

If the attempt to make children's sports safe and successful is a high-wire act, then I hope this book will serve as a balancing pole. It's my sincere hope that I can help you provide your children with a sports experience they will take with them into adulthood — along with a lifetime interest in health and fitness.

Acknowledgments

I am pleased to acknowledge the contributions of several persons to this book. My thanks go to Mark Jenkins, who helped translate complex scientific concepts into language understood by the layperson; to Julie Power, my research assistant, who spent long hours typing and retyping the manuscript and retrieving long-lost papers and documents from my filing cabinets; and to the numerous colleagues who assisted me during the past decade in conducting pioneering research in the field of pediatric and adolescent sports medicine. I am indebted to my wife, Anne, whose patience during the time-consuming process of preparing this work is greatly appreciated. This book would not have been possible without the vision of my friend and teacher Dr. John Hall, chairman of orthopedics at Boston Children's Hospital, who in 1974 gave me his permission and blessing to organize the world's first clinic to study the special problems of young athletes.

1

• • • • •

Children's Sports:
Questions and Answers

As director of sports medicine at Children's Hospital in Boston, I'm responsible for the assessment, treatment, and rehabilitation of thousands of young athletes each year. And for every sports-injured youngster, there's a concerned parent with a list of sports questions as long as your arm. I encourage these questions. An informed parent is better able to help prevent future injuries and to help me in facilitating the child's rehabilitation.

However, many of these parents ask similar questions. For this reason, in 1986 I began writing a column for *Children* magazine to answer many of the common questions. Some of these issues are addressed in the following chapters, but with the kind permission of the publishers of *Children*, I'm reproducing a selection of the published questions here, along with a few others.

What is the difference between free play and organized sports?

Free play is unconstrained, undirected playing, often in competitive games that involve physical activity. The primary motivation is usually fun. In free play the children themselves pick the teams and set the rules to fit the situation. In organized sports children participate in a specific individual or team sport with fixed rules and playing times. Often the training for these sports is a regimented series of regular practices under adult supervision. While children's free play has been around since the dawn of mankind, organized sports for children are relatively new. The first effective organized sports program outside of schools at the community level was the Little League organization, which expanded shortly after World War II. Community-based leagues now exist for almost every sport you can think of.

Which sport should my child play?

The answer to this question can be very difficult or quite easy. Perhaps the most important criterion is that the sport should be one the child is interested in and enjoys. An important factor in your child's enjoyment will be the quality of the instruction, which may vary widely from one community to another. A hockey program in one town may be very well supervised and taught in such a way that the children truly have a good time. Usually competition isn't the be-all and end-all of such a program. But in the next town the hockey program may be quite the opposite, with officials and coaches who do not set good examples of sportsmanship and enjoyment of the game. In the long run the child will learn bad habits and bad hockey in such a program. Therefore it's important to research the sports program in which your child will become involved. Try to speak to parents and children who have been involved in the program to find what their experiences have been. For more on choosing a sport, see Chapter 2.

Are some children naturally unathletic?

In all my years dealing with children, I can't say I've encountered one who couldn't develop skills and proficiency in at least one sport. One major development in this country over the past few years has been the diversification of sports for children. In the past most schools would offer only three organized sports at the most, usually baseball, football, and basketball. Now it is quite common to see as many as twelve to fourteen different activities available to both boys and girls.

This diversification, in conjunction with the development of sports such as martial arts at the community and club level, has made it possible for every child to participate in an organized sport or fitness activity. Interestingly, children who are brought to me because their parents think they are "unathletic" seem to make the most progress in coordination, strength, and flexibility when they join a martial arts program. This suggests that the coaching in these programs is very good, and that the instructors have the patience to work with all sorts of children. It is always immensely gratifying for me to see children who are initially discouraged about their supposed lack of athletic prowess evolve into fit, coordinated, and confident young persons as a result of their involvement in martial arts.

After bandaging my twelve-year-old for what seems like the twelfth time this month, I'm wondering if he could be injury-prone?

Yes, he could be. Children with deficits in strength, range, or flexibility are particularly vulnerable to falls, pulled muscles, and other mishaps. Your child may have tight hamstring muscles or a weak lower back and pelvis. Perhaps he's more sedentary and doesn't "work" his muscles as much as his friends who are always climbing trees and playing soccer (see Chapter 3). Or a recent growth spurt may have created dramatic tightness in his muscles because the bones grew more rapidly. (Injuries are discussed in Chapters 4 and 5.) In either case, when the school gym teacher assigns your child to the relay team or when he joins in a neighborhood game of chase, injuries such as a pulled muscle may occur.

The best way to help an injury-prone child play safely is to improve his flexibility. Get him walking (ideally, with you) for forty minutes at a time, three times a week. Teach him some stretches to do regularly. YMCAs often have excellent stretching and fitness classes for young people. In Chapter 8 you'll find a series of flexibility exercises that will benefit any child.

Another reason for a child to seem injury-prone is psychological in nature. Kids under great social stress, because of divorce, a recent family move or a relative's death, for instance, seem to be more vulnerable to injury.

My oldest child was our state's high school swimming champion last year. Now our youngest, who's nine and has asthma, wants to follow her sister and start training. Is it safe for an asthmatic child to participate in sports?

Yes, it's safe and even beneficial if certain guidelines are followed. Your daughter chose the best sport for someone with asthma to pursue. Swimming, with its moist environment, actually seems to improve the condition. And swimming builds endurance slowly. You need to be more concerned about an asthmatic child in sports such as wrestling, track, or baseball, which involve sudden, hard-on-the-body changes from inactivity to activity. Having asthma doesn't rule out these sports, but there is a greater chance of an attack (sudden labored breathing) occurring.

To make sports as safe as they are fun for your child, be sure your doctor is following her condition and knows what activity she is participating in. Be sure the event is supervised, and make teachers aware of her condition. Have your child carry any asthma medication that has been prescribed for her at all times. Beware of colds and emotional upsets, which can cause flare-ups.

Two encouraging notes: exercise often decreases the amount of medication a child needs to take for asthma, and most asthma gets better as a child grows older. It may even go away completely. For more on sports for children with chronic illnesses, see Chapter 12.

When my daughter is injured during a field hockey game, I sometimes worry that her coach sends her back in too quickly. (She's the leading scorer.) Are there any guidelines on when it's safe — and when it's foolish — to let an injured child go back in?

Definitely. And it's important for you to be aware of these guidelines, because some coaches are not adequately trained to handle sports emergencies. First, in the case of an injury to the head, neck, back, or eyes the child should be removed from the game and get prompt medical attention. No one can pinpoint the seriousness of such an injury from the sidelines.

There's a simple five-minute rule for four kinds of injuries: having the wind knocked out; swelling or hampered range of motion in a joint such as the elbow, hip, or knee; lingering abdominal pain; or a persistent limp. If one of these injuries occurs, your child should wait five minutes. If the problem goes away, it's probably safe to continue playing. If pain persists, a doctor should check her immediately. For more safety guidelines, see Chapters 4 and 5.

Should I let my child quit a team?

If a child comes home and declares that he is going to quit the team, I believe it's extremely important for the parent to explore the child's reasons in detail. Often the initial reason given isn't the real one, and the child may actually be in a stressful team situation without consciously realizing it. It's been my experience that having a parent intervene by changing the child's team or coach may alter the situation dramatically without the child having to leave the program. In other situations the sport may be one that the child simply doesn't enjoy, and here the child's wish must be respected. The parent should emphasize the importance of sports and fitness and help the child find a different activity.

My husband is encouraging our son to go out for football because he says sports build character. Is there any evidence that that's true? From what I've seen of the football coach, who has an almost fanatic need to win, I don't think he's the right person to be building my son's character.

This has long been a controversial question. In fact, a whole field of study, called the sociology of sports, looks primarily at the arguments on both sides of the character-building debate. My answer is that sports don't necessarily do this. Some evidence suggests that team sports such as football actually build *conformity,* not character. The answer really depends on one thing: how the coach structures the team.

A well-organized team can teach good work habits, a sense of responsibility, and fair play. When these qualities aren't a coach's priority, however, a child's character might even be eroded.

Two youth hockey teams here in the Boston area are a perfect example. Team A trains to develop strength, agility, and team effort. The players generally become self-disciplined adults with a keen sense of sportsmanship. Team B is noted for being particularly nasty and violent. Players from this group often turn out to be less than model citizens.

A very interesting study of youth soccer programs in the Los Angeles area found that coaches had more impact on kids' sense of self-worth than either parents or teammates did! What to do, then, when a person with great responsibility for shaping your child's values has a whiplike temper, doesn't play fairly, and lives for the big win? You can try to counter the coach's bad influence by discussing with your child attitudes and behaviors you don't want him to adopt. But you'd be better off switching your son to another team, especially if he is under twelve, when children are most impressionable. You need to be a good watchdog for your child when he asks to join a particular team. Observe a practice, not a game. A less-than-sterling coach may be "on good behavior" in front of a bleacherful of parents. Find out if the coach has had training in teaching children, and ask parents of older children what they thought of the coach's style and character. Much more on children's sports psychology can be found in Chapter 6.

My son is on the swim team at school, and a few weeks ago they got a new coach who used to coach college swimmers. He told my son's team he was going to turn them into state champions, but I think he's pushing the children to exhaustion. Should I be concerned? Is it possible for a child to get too much exercise?

It is, and we see this all the time. It's called overtraining. When children are playing by themselves, running around the neighborhood, and climbing trees, there's rarely a danger of overexertion. But organized sports carry a real potential for problems when kids are trained to — and often beyond — their limits.

In individual performance sports, such as swimming, gymnastics, and figure skating, overzealous coaching is a particular problem. Overtraining seems to be on the rise at every level. Ten years ago the average member of a college swim team swam 5,000 yards a day while training. Today, nine-year-olds are being told to swim this same distance.

Have you noticed any changes in your son? Sleeplessness, weight loss, irritability, problems at school, and loss of appetite are common signs that the exercise has gone from being helpful to being hurtful. At this point injury and emotional burnout are likely to hit. If you feel your son is suffering, you should see whether the coach is willing to pull back; if he is not, ask your son if he wants to pull out.

My daughter's friends found out that they were too young to join the local health clubs, so they started their own "aerobics club." Each girl bought a workout video, and they exercise to them every night. Are video workouts effective and safe?

Your daughter and her friends have taken up one of today's most popular forms of exercise. But while aerobic dance can be an excellent way to build cardiovascular fitness, it's not as innocuous as previously thought. This is especially true when home videocassettes are involved. We've seen a lot of injuries, most of which could easily have been avoided.

The biggest problem with video workouts is that there's no instructor in the room with you. In a class the teacher can look at you, see what you're doing wrong, and correct improper moves before you injure a muscle, joint, or ligament. The instructor can also make sure you do enough warm-up stretching to get your muscles ready for action — something too many people skimp on or skip altogether.

Also, consider why you buy a particular exercise video. You're impressed by the star's body and stamina, which are generally better and stronger than yours. And there's almost always a show-off factor: the exercises are repeated many times and performed at high speed. (If the stars performed at your level, you wouldn't be inspired.) Unfortunately, the average video workout pace is much too fast for most of us to perform safely. We struggle and strain to keep up, and that's how we get injured.

The following guidelines apply to people of any age who use exercise videocassettes:

- Start each session with at least ten minutes of slow, total-body stretching. If the warm-up is too brief, press the pause button and keep stretching.
- Individualize the program to your fitness level and your abilities. Don't work yourself into a frenzy trying to crank out two

hundred sit-ups just because the video says to. If you start out with twenty, great.

• Avoid sudden jarring movements. Your joints should never feel as if they're being bounced. The new low-impact aerobics are much smarter.

My fifth-grader recently asked me why all the sports teams at school are either "all boys" or "all girls." Good question! Is there some reason why both sexes shouldn't compete together?

Our society has never been big on mixing the sexes in sports. Look at the Olympics: only one sport — equestrian riding — combines men and women. It's my guess that sports stay segregated because participants *want* it that way. Most boys and girls get more enjoyment from competing against their own sex. This may not be true of young children, but it certainly is of older ones. Size attributes may be one reason.

Up until sixth grade there's no significant difference in size and strength between boys and girls. (This is one reason why Little League baseball has allowed some girls to join the boys.) But when puberty goes into full swing, most boys become bigger (and usually stronger) than most girls.

Scientific experiments have shown that if men and women together run the hundred-yard dash and the ten-kilometer race, not even the most elite female runners would be able to beat the top male athletes. That may sound unfair, but it's true. Look at the most recent Boston Marathon. The top male runner finished in two hours and ten minutes. The top female took fourteen minutes longer to complete the race. Whether this phenomenon exists because males are physically better suited for all-out competition or because they benefit from better training and coaching throughout their lives hasn't been proven to anyone's satisfaction yet.

At any rate, most boys and girls want to compete at their own level, and thus don't often seek to play on the same team. But the occasional child who wants to break tradition shouldn't be discouraged from doing so, provided her physical attributes are appropriate for the sport.

Do athletes really get sick less often than people who are out of shape, or is this just a sports myth?

It's never been well documented, but a number of observers have suggested that improving your physical condition improves your general health and increases your resistance to common viral illnesses. Some experts believe that when the body is stressed by conditioning exercises, it secretes certain natural hormones, called adrenocorticals, which help us resist infection. So far, most of the evidence for this link has been found in athletic people who have been injured or are having elective surgery; they appear to recover better from the physical trauma of injury and have a greater resistance to infection after surgery than nonathletic people. But the answer to this question has been difficult to pin down scientifically.

Every time my son gets ready for Little League practice, he complains of having a stomachache and "not feeling good," just as he did when he first went off to school. Is it time to take him out of the league?

Your son may not be able to put his finger on exactly what is bothering him, so he has developed somatic complaints — the familiar stomachache, for instance. This, I'm sure you're aware, is how kids subconsciously attempt to avoid stressful situations.

Your son may be feeling the pressure of organized sports. The competitiveness of some of these systems can be a real problem for many kids. Another possibility is that your son just doesn't like the sport as much as he thinks *you* want him to. He could be unhappy with the way the practices are run, the coach's style, or something a teammate is doing. It's important not to minimize the problem. Minor complaints can warn of impending injuries. Children who are under stress seem to have a greater incidence of injury. Your son probably will appreciate some frank discussions about his worries. Ask him if he truly likes playing baseball and emphasize that it's fine with you if he decides he'd rather be doing something else. You may want to explore other options, such as changing teams or practicing together to improve a weak skill.

Should parents coach their own children?

The rise of community-based sports programs has meant that it is commonplace for parents to be coaching their own children. That situation can be a delicate one, but I've seen it handled very well in many cases. The parent-coach must be very careful to make sure that absolute fairness is used in selecting teams and positions on teams when his own child is involved. In addition, he should make it clear to the child in private that no preference will be given. It's been my experience that when these simple guidelines are followed, there are relatively few problems.

I don't think my son should go off to gymnastic meets on an empty stomach. But he says food will hamper his performance, and he would rather eat when he comes home. When is the best time for an athlete to eat — before or after an event?

Here's the strategy that research has shown works best: four hours before an event, your child should eat a fairly light meal of complex carbohydrates, such as pasta, cereals, or whole-grain breads. "Carbos" are easily digested and are readily converted to glycogen, which is stored in muscles and used for energy. (One theory claims that a higher intake of carbos throughout the week will result in twice the amount of stored muscle glycogen.) Eating four hours before the event allows the body to concentrate on digestion. If other muscles are called into action right after a meal, the body has to give short shrift to either the exerted muscles or the full stomach. When the stomach gets shortchanged, cramps and diarrhea are possible.

Your budding athlete should stay away from foods high in fat and protein before a sporting event. If the image of thick, juicy steaks on a training table comes to mind, be aware that this tradition has given way to smarter, lighter eating. The only thing steak ever does for an athlete is stay in the stomach too long. Also on the save-it-for-later list are dairy products, which can trigger diarrhea during the event (especially if the event requires endurance), and candy bars. Candy may raise blood sugar levels initially, but it eventually produces a sharp *drop* in those levels.

Here's another smart nutrition move people don't always remember: drink lots of water. Fluid intake is important for endurance events, such as cross-country running or biking, to prevent dehydration. And if the weather is warm or humid, athletes in *any* sport should drink plenty of water. Other good pre-sport nourishments include bananas, which are easy to digest, and noncarbonated fruit juices.

After the practice or competition, anything in the kitchen is fair game. Your child may not feel hungry until an hour or so after practice or competition: exercise often has a short-term appetite-suppressing effect. Digestion is easier after the game because the tension and anxiety are gone. See Chapter 9 for much more on nutrition for the child athlete.

Our son is a tremendous athlete. Should we be doing something special for him?

I've seen many extremely gifted young athletes get injured because of overly aggressive coaching. When an amateur coach encounters a particularly gifted athlete, there's a natural tendency to increase the workload, which may increase the stress level on the child. Sometimes overuse injuries occur, which can ruin a fine athletic future. At the very least the child may suffer increasing psychological stress. Parents of an athletically gifted child must be particularly cautious to ensure that he isn't being pushed too hard by a coach interested in promoting himself and the program at the expense of the child. Parents must act as an ombudsman for their child in this situation.

Our school has decided to hire a full-time trainer. Is that a good idea? What's the difference between a trainer and a coach?

Hiring a school trainer is a good, cost-effective way to make sports safer for kids. Every school with an athletic program from the junior-high level up, should have a full-time trainer on staff. The position is one of the best developments that has come along in school sports.

The trainer ideally should be part of a triumvirate, along with the team doctor and the coach. The trainer handles first aid, teaches injury prevention and proper nutrition, makes initial assessments of injuries, and determines whether or not a doctor's visit is necessary. The trainer also helps with any therapy an injured player needs before going back into a game. Trainers cannot prescribe medications, but they can administer ice, heat, elevation, and other first-aid measures.

To become a school trainer, a person must major in athletic training in college and take a certifying exam. (Look for the initials A.T.C., for Athletic Training Certified, after the name.) Or she can enter the field as a registered physical therapist with 1,000 hours of on-the-job training.

My son is a great baseball player. Unfortunately, nine other boys are even better, and he only made the second team. Do you think it would bolster his confidence to switch to another sport, such as track, where he could be more active and really show what he's made of?

Sure, second string can be disappointing at times. Too often the second-string player gets off the bench only during the last few minutes of a runaway game, when there's no chance of the other team catching up.

But if you think about it, you'll see how much your son can gain from the second-string experience. First, your son must enjoy being on the team, or he probably would have quit by now. He likes the sport and enjoys being part of it all. Don't forget, along with the scheduled games, there are countless practice sessions (which provide plenty of physical activity), away-game bus trips, banquets, and more, all the way down to the quiet thrills of wearing the uniform, being in the yearbook team photo, and earning a letter at the season's end.

If you think about it, your son *is* showing what he's made of: strong character. His name may not be the one the crowd chants, but he's contributing to a team effort anyway. His self-confidence grows when he realizes he can be valuable even if he's not a star.

He's also learning there are some things no one is able to change, such as body size and skill level, but that anyone can both accept and live with limitations. This kind of self-acceptance isn't always easy for people. He can certainly still enjoy his chosen sport and work to the best of his ability. And while the term "team spirit" may be a cliché, it's something he'll always need in his family, work, and personal life.

One other note: just because his baseball talent falls a little short now doesn't mean he won't improve later, say, in college. Team stars are most valuable when they are team *players* first, and your son's experiences on the second string are likely to enhance his sense of teamwork all around.

Are injuries more likely to occur in certain sports than in others?

Interestingly, the potential for injury in certain children's sports seems to be most closely related to the way the sport is directed and the intensity of the training. Although high school football has a high rate of injury, in Pop Warner football, which is for children below the age of fourteen, injuries are very rare because the quality of supervision is very high. On the other hand, soccer, which has a reputation for being a safe sport for both sexes, has been shown to have a high injury rate, particularly among younger children. In this age group, preparing a child for the sport, teaching the fundamentals, and training at a reasonable pace will minimize the risk of injury in any sport. The exception to this is boxing, which I strongly discourage for children younger than fourteen years.

My father still suffers from a knee injury he got playing basketball in high school. My daughter knows this, but she wants to play field hockey anyway. I'm worried she'll end up the same way. Is there any way to prevent knee injuries?

Short of skipping athletics altogether, nothing can guarantee against knee injuries. Knees are the most frequently hurt area in almost every sport. You do need to be concerned, since some types of knee injuries can bother a person for the rest of her life. Other types heal (or are healed by surgery), and the athlete is as good as new. The part of the knee that's hurt determines the severity of the injury.

Injuries to this vulnerable joint happen in two ways. *Single macrotrauma*, or acute injury, is the result of a single incident, such as being hit in the knee or twisting it the wrong way. *Repetitive microtrauma* is the so-called overuse injury, an ache or irritation that develops over a period of time.

There are three types of knee injuries:

Ligamentous injury. Ligaments run from bone to bone to hold the knee together. A blow to the knee can cause this trauma, but the most common cause is twisting, or "cutting," the sudden change of direction often called for in football, basketball, skiing, soccer, lacrosse, and field hockey. This is the most serious accident, often requiring immediate surgery, which may or may not be successful.

Internal derangement, or torn cartilage. The injury is to either the articular cartilage, which runs over the surface of the knee joint and resembles the glistening white cartilage you find when you cut up a chicken, or to the meniscal cartilage, which is like two half washers that fit on both sides of the knee. When people say they have had arthroscopic surgery, it is usually cartilage that needed fixing. Two to three weeks after surgery these people are able to start running again.

Extensor mechanism injury. The extensor mechanism is the system that enables you to straighten your lower leg. It includes the kneecap, the tendon over it, the places where the tendon inserts into the bone, and the thigh muscle above the kneecap. Unless you're talking about a broken patella (the kneecap), overuse is the most common cause of trouble in the extensor mechanism. You'll recognize this in the athlete who, after a couple of weeks of training, starts to feel an ache in her knee. It hurts when she sits in one place for awhile or bothers her when she goes up and down stairs. In this initial stage, just the kneecap may be irritated. But if the injury is left untreated, the articular cartilage can be damaged. Then you've got a more serious condition called chondromalacia. Extensor mechanism injury is the number-one problem we see in junior-high kids today.

A few precautions can help protect the knees. I can't stress enough the importance of a good pre-sports physical by a physician who's really interested in sports medicine. He can look for clues that your child is predisposed to knee injuries: knock-knees, bowlegs, or poorly positioned kneecaps, for instance. This kind of diagnosis won't necessarily consign her to the chess or golf team. But she may need to start a specific exercise program to strengthen the inside of her knee and stretch the outside, wear arch supports, or approach the sport at a slower pace than other youngsters.

Another critical factor in protecting knees is regular strength training on Nautilus-type equipment. Sports medicine physicians now realize that strength training not only improves muscles, it strengthens ligaments and bones, too. Leg-building exercises include thigh extensions and presses, knee flexes, and adductions and abductions. The key to performing these successfully is to proceed slowly and to use a fairly heavy weight.

Since your child has chosen a running sport, be sure she steers clear of knee-mauling hills and doesn't always run on super-hard surfaces, especially early on. A knee brace made of neoprene (similar to wet-suit material) and designed with the kneecap area uncovered, may take some of the pressure off the patella and prevent irritation. If the problem becomes severe, a sports doctor may prescribe a pneumatic brace such as the ones pioneered by AIRCAST. You can find this type of brace in drugstores and sporting goods stores. Refer to Chapters 4 and 5 for much more on injury prevention and treatment.

After my daughter complained of an aching shin for several days, her gymnastics coach told her she might have a stress fracture. What could have caused this, and what should be done about it?

Repetitive pounding can create a tiny bone crack called a stress fracture. The jumping and flipping your daughter does in gymnastic events make her a prime candidate for this injury.

Stress fractures, originally called "march fractures," were first noticed during wartime, when normally sedentary folk such as bankers were called into duty and made to march for miles every day. Years ago stress fractures were rare in children. But in today's competitive sports and heavy training schedules many young athletes have been sidelined with the condition. Gymnasts aren't the only ones at high risk. Sprinters, jumpers, and long-distance runners are vulnerable because of the jarring their legs receive.

A low-grade ache or pain in a bone is usually the only clue to the presence of a stress fracture. At this point the fracture can't even be seen on an X ray. With proper care it can heal on its own. If the pain is ignored and the jarring activity continues, however, the bone will go through a cycle of partial healing and refracturing. After about three weeks of this, a painful lump will form at the fracture site. If the condition remains untreated, there is a *slight* chance the crack will deepen and the bone will break all the way through. One young runner I treated had had knee pain for five weeks but was told by his coach to "stick it out, it's probably just tendinitis." Five weeks later his leg broke.

An accurate and prompt diagnosis is therefore crucial. If there's an unexplained pain in an arm or leg or even the pelvis, hip, or knee, try icing the area for twenty minutes a day for seven to ten days. If the pain still hangs on, see a doctor.

Treatment may be as simple as resting the injured area for several weeks. "Rest" is a relative term here: if running led to the fracture, it may be all right to switch to a less jarring activity like swimming. Some cases require a few weeks on crutches, however. A cast or splint could also be necessary.

To prevent further bone cracking in the injured area (or even in a new spot), it's important to strengthen the muscle around the fracture. This will help the body to withstand the shock of the activity. Finally, to lessen the forces on the leg, special impact-absorbing shoe inserts may be prescribed. Overuse injuries such as stress fractures are covered in depth in Chapter 5.

No cheerleading for my daughter — she wants to join the football team! My wife and I don't know what to think, but the coach sure does. He said girls' bodies can't take that kind of punishment, and he refused to let her try out. Is he right?

Both boys and girls who have developed strength, flexibility, and conditioning can play football safely. It's when you talk about them playing *together* that the issue gets tricky.

If your daughter is tall and solid (five foot eight, 180 pounds, for example), lifts weights, and practices stretching and flexibility exercises, there's no reason for her not to play football (or any other contact sport, for that matter) with boys. Scientific evidence has made no clear determination that she'd be more injury-prone than any boy on the team.

If she is smaller than that, the story is different. It's inadvisable for a girl to play contact sports with boys who are taller, bigger framed, and more developed physically. (For that matter, it's inadvisable for a smaller-built *boy* to compete with bigger teammates.) The average woman doesn't develop the size or strength necessary for avoiding injury in coed contact sports.

One plan that does work well is for women to play contact sports with each other. Women's football leagues, even at the high school level, have been very successful. And a new sport on the scene, women's rugby, is rapidly gaining popularity. Women can safely play rugby with just as much heavy contact as men if they are competing against similar body types.

If you think your daughter is a good candidate for the boys' football team, have a sports medicine physician give her a pre-sports physical. The doctor will check her general health as well as gauge her "sports-specific" fitness level. Even if she is fast on her feet, she could be lacking in the upper-body strength crucial for competing safely. If this is the case, she should undertake a weight-lifting program before participating, or consider a different sport.

Should a child who is not performing well in school participate in athletics?

I think parents should be extremely cautious about eliminating sports when the child isn't doing well academically. It's much more important to pursue why the child is having problems in his academic subjects and not use the denial of sports activity as a punishment. However, I've encountered some youngsters who devote excessive time and effort to sports, often to the detriment of academic performance. They, and their parents as well, have totally lost their perspective on academics and sports. A child who gets up at 4:30 A.M. to make a 6:00 A.M. swimming or hockey practice is losing sleeping time that is essential for growth and without which he can't perform well in the classroom.

My late-blooming son is getting the tar knocked out of him by bigger boys on the football team. He thinks he'll fare better if he "bulks up" by lifting weights. His coach, however, says weightlifting will interfere with the growth spurt he's anxiously awaiting. Could this happen?

Not for the reason the coach is probably thinking of. One popular sports myth concerns what are called *growth plates* at the ends of bones, the areas at which all bone growth takes place. Some people believe, incorrectly, that lifting weights puts so much pressure on these plates that a child's growth will be stunted. What weightlifting *can* do, recent research shows, is strengthen the bones and surrounding ligaments.

Improper use of weights, however, is another story. Growth plates can fracture because of bad lifting technique, as in the overhead lifting done in the "military press" and "squats." For growing children, other lifts may strain the lower back or knees. A fractured growth plate is one way growth could be stunted. This potential danger is why some experts don't want children lifting weights. With proper instruction and supervision, though, it can be a beneficial exercise for children. Strength training is covered in depth in Chapter 8.

Is it wise for my daughter to keep going to track and field practice with a cold? Will exercise really "sweat the illness out," as they say, or will she just end up feeling worse?

If your daughter just has a slight cold, she can probably safely continue to train. She may not turn out any "personal bests" at this time, but she won't harm herself. However, if she has a viral infection with fever, she *should not* perform any kind of aerobic activity until she's better.

A growing concern among sports medicine specialists is that when the body is fighting a viral infection and doing aerobic work, there is an increased chance of cardiac problems. Viral illnesses may increase the heart's "irritability" by interfering with its electrical currents. This increases the chance of cardiac arrhythmias, or palpitations. (Once the athlete has recovered from the virus, however, no threat remains.)

As for sweating out an illness, the only benefit some people find is that exercise "opens them up" a bit if they're congested, helping to loosen and drain secretions. This result is most frequently reported by swimmers, but in their case the humidity that goes with indoor pools may be a more important factor.

My daughter's arm was broken in a basketball game, and she just had the cast removed. Does her arm need babying for awhile, or should she try to do as much as possible with it?

Babying the newly mended arm isn't necessary, but rehabilitation is. Your daughter's bone is probably as strong as ever if X rays have shown that it has healed. But remember, X rays can't show muscle strength. The supporting muscles and ligaments have lost a considerable amount of strength, flexibility, and range of motion from being confined in a cast, and they stand a greater chance of being injured.

Your daughter should do exercises supervised by a physical therapist until the mended arm is judged to be within 5 percent of the strength of the uninjured arm. The range of motion of the joint near the fracture site should be the same as for the opposite arm. Swimming and bicycling are smart ways to ease back into sports training.

My ten-year-old son is planning to try out for Little League baseball or football. Should he have a physical first? If so, what should it entail?

A good pre-sports physical should assess your son's overall physical fitness and determine whether he has any diseases, injuries, or problems that might prevent him from participating safely in sports. The doctor should examine his eyes, check the heart and kidneys, and evaluate cardiovascular and musculoskeletal fitness. He should make sure your son has complete range of motion of the head, neck, shoulders, back, hips, knees, and ankles. The doctor should ask for a complete health history to identify potential problems or risks. Certain conditions, such as an impaired organ or only one kidney, eye, or testicle, for example, may disqualify a child from playing certain sports.

Nowadays the pre-sports physical should be specific to the sport. If a child is interested in gymnastics, the doctor should make sure that the hamstrings are not too tight. If he is interested in football, the doctor will measure his strength to see whether he can withstand the rigors of the sport.

The pre-sports physical provides an opportunity to assess children and counsel them on an appropriate sport. If your child has his heart set on a certain sport yet has a physical weakness, the doctor may be able to give him supplemental exercises so he can participate eventually. If the weakness can't be corrected, your child may have to pick a different sport.

It's very important for your child to have a physical if he is seriously concentrating on a sport and training at least three times a week. The earlier the evaluation, the better his chance of avoiding problems later. For much more on the pre-sports physical, refer to Chapter 7.

I never know whether to apply heat or cold to a pulled muscle. The next time my daughter comes home with one, I want to get it right. How should a pulled muscle be handled?

The best way to treat a pulled muscle, properly referred to as a muscle strain, is to apply ice to the injured area and rest it until the pain and swelling have gone away. When muscle tissue is torn, it becomes inflamed and tight. To reduce the inflammation, apply ice — twelve minutes on and twenty to thirty minutes off — for a period of three to seven days, depending on the seriousness of the injury. A useful technique for ice massage is to fill a plastic-foam cup with water and freeze it, then cut off the top edge of the cup and massage the injured area with the exposed ice.

After the pain and swelling have subsided, you can start rehabilitating the area with gentle exercise and movement. Don't let your child do too much too soon, or she will risk reinjuring the muscle. Be patient: it may take up to three or four weeks to restore strength and motion to the area. Treatment of injuries is covered in Chapter 4.

How can a handicapped child participate in sports?

Our society has seen tremendous growth and development in sports for physically impaired children. As with an able-bodied child, it's extremely important to respect the handicapped child's wishes and desires. The parent may gently encourage him to participate in a physical activity, but it's essential that the child determine the sport and the level of intensity he wishes to become involved in. While physical activity can have a tremendous positive impact on emotional and physical development, a negative experience can be devastating.

2

• • • • •

Should Your Child
Play Sports?

While driving through the suburbs on a sunny spring afternoon, you chance upon an emerald-green patch of manicured grass upon which thirty youngsters in pristine white uniforms are learning the mysteries of that most American of pastimes, baseball. A timeless portrait of American youth, right?

Think again. Organized sports are such a prominent feature of American folk culture that we are inclined to imagine that Little League baseball and Pop Warner football arrived on these shores with the *Mayflower*. But in fact, organized sports for children became a part of the fabric of American society only after World War II. Only in the past quarter century have they become a ubiquitous part of the American scene. Before that time, free play and sandlot sports dominated the leisure time of American children. The change in the character of children's play from unstructured to organized doesn't please everyone. When I attend conferences I hear many of my colleagues waxing nostalgic about the bygone days of free play and decrying the rise of organized sports. "Those were the days" is their theme.

Frankly, I find the debate over the relative merits of free play versus organized sports irrelevant. Like those who miss the horse and carriage, many people mourn the passing of the old ways of play. But we must realize that several profound changes in our society have contributed to the organization of children's sports, among them the limited number of recreational facilities, the progressive loss of open space and vacant lots in cities and suburbs, and the decrease in spontaneous neighborhood activities. The American family structure has changed; separation and divorce are common, and in many families both parents work outside the home. These changes have made organized sports an attractive option for many parents who simply can't keep an eye on what the kids are up to. Our lives have become so busy and structured that organized programs fit well into our compartmentalized existence.

The Rewards of Sports

There's no question in my mind that well-organized athletic programs can provide a safe, wholesome environment where our children can enjoy their spare time. Goodness knows there are too many negative temptations available to our children. I'm not talking only about illegal temptations like drugs, alcohol, and unsafe, unwise sexual experiences. There are also television, video games, junk food, and fancy toys, which are perfectly legal as well as perfectly terrible for this nation's youngsters. You can extol the virtues of educational television, interactive video games, and brain-building toys as much as you want, but I've seen too many casualties of such modern technology to be impressed. I'm talking about fat children with a list of heart-disease risk factors as long as their arms; I'm talking about children so weak they can barely do one sit-up; I'm talking about children whose muscles are so "tight" they can't touch their knees. These are kids who have been denied the chance to participate in fitness-building activities. Far too many of our youngsters are missing out on

Potential Benefits of Playing Sports

●

Builds health fitness
Teaches good health fitness habits
Teaches basic sports skills
Teaches healthy competition
Develops self-esteem
Develops friendships
Provides pleasure

the physical activity their bodies need to reach their full potential, not to mention the rewarding experiences sports provide that help them develop into fully formed adults.

Health Fitness

"Health fitness" is the healthy state achieved through regular exercise. Its three components are heart-lung endurance (cardiovascular fitness), strength and flexibility (musculoskeletal fitness), and a good ratio of body fat to muscle (nutritional fitness). All three components are essential for children's short- and long-term good health. Kids who exercise regularly have bigger hearts, more muscle mass, less fatty tissue, stronger bones, and more flexible joints. Being fit in childhood helps people fight off a host of diseases in later life, including heart disease, back pain, and osteoporosis. Fit children are far less likely to be injured in sports than youngsters who aren't in shape. Recent evidence also suggests that regular exercise helps youngsters' academic performance; this is the "healthy mind in a healthy body" concept that has been with us since the time of the ancient Greeks. Health fitness is vital for us all — children, adults, and the elderly. I'm strongly in favor of youngsters balancing sports like football and baseball, which don't really promote fitness, with health fitness builders like swimming, running, soccer, cycling, and strength training with weights. These activities keep kids in shape and provide opportunities for lifetime participation. Chapter 3 discusses health fitness for children in more depth.

Good Health Fitness Habits

Those who play sports in childhood are very likely to continue to do so as adults. We get used to feeling good and strive to keep feeling that way. For that reason it's very important that children learn good health fitness habits early in life. In addition to encouraging kids to exercise, sports can teach why exercise is so important. For example, young swimmers can learn to read their pulses — they get a huge kick out of this — and from a very early age they can understand that maintaining a high pulse rate for at least twenty minutes three times a week is a good way to guarantee the long-term health of their hearts. By the same token, children must learn the life-threatening — this is no exaggeration — consequences of a sedentary lifestyle. Once again, it is very important that we promote the health fitness–building sports that can be played through life. That way, when baseball, football, basketball, and ice hockey are no longer available or appealing to them in adulthood, our kids will have a background in activities like cycling, jogging, and swimming to help them keep in shape.

Sports Skills

Children love learning new skills. It's a natural part of growing up to want to absorb as much knowledge as possible and use it in different situations. Having new knowledge makes kids feel more confident and self-assured. Sports skills are especially important because they are tools for staying fit and healthy throughout life as well as for effective participation in childhood activities. As far as I'm concerned, the more skills your child can learn, the better. The youngster who learns to play baseball, squash, soccer, and basketball and is taught to swim, cycle, and jog properly has a packed toolbox of sports skills that can be used throughout life. I'm much more interested in having children learn five different sports than getting them to specialize in just one. The rise of the young specialist athlete explains in large part the increasing incidence of overuse injuries. At the same time, it's extremely important that children be properly coached. Incorrectly learning a skill such as baseball pitching can lead to serious injury.

Healthy Competition

Children love to compete. Despite what some critics say, competition between kids didn't start with organized sports. It's been around since our ancestors were living in caves. What sports can do is teach children to compete fairly, to try their hardest, to congratulate the winners if they lose, and to accept victory gracefully if they win. This is the old-fashioned notion of sportsmanship, which I feel has been overlooked in recent times. Children exposed to healthy competition will soon learn that the reason they play sports isn't to win at all costs, but to strive to win by playing as hard as they can within the boundaries of a set of rules. I truly believe that when left to their own devices, children are much more interested in competing than in winning. These are not the same thing. Just watch kids playing a fierce game of soccer among themselves, and then ask them what the score is.

Most of the time they won't know! Most important, children who learn to play hard and fairly will take this approach with them into other areas of their adult lives.

Self-Esteem

One of the most important things sports can do is build self-esteem. Children have to grow emotionally as well as physically, and sports can help them develop a positive self-image and become much more confident. It isn't necessary to be the star of the team to be successful in sports. Any child who feels as if she is contributing to the team effort will learn self-esteem. The goals set for each child should be realistic; as they achieve these goals they understand that they are developing as athletes. Don't forget, if your child is having difficulty in a team sport like baseball or football, you should encourage him to take up an activity that allows greater scope for competing against himself — jogging, cycling, strength training, or swimming, for example.

Friendship

One of the great rewards of sports is socializing. Sports give kids the chance to be with a large group of peers in a stimulating environment. The more sports your child plays, the more friends she has the chance to make. It is a testament to the power of sports that these friendships often last through life. Children should be encouraged to make friends on opposing teams as well as their own. When a barbecue is held after a Little League game, the kids have an opportunity to get to know one another personally. That's where the true spirit of youth sports can be found. Children learn to leave rivalries on the field and discover that their opponents are kids like themselves who just want to have fun in sports.

Pleasure

Ah, fun! For kids, this is the number-one reason to play sports. I suspect that many adults have forgotten how much fun we had in sports when we were kids. And many have forgotten *how* we had that fun. We impose adult measurements of success — trophies, uniforms, leagues, and so on. The rationale is that if we don't give kids these things, they'll quit sports. But that's simply not true. Children were playing among themselves long before anybody invented trophies or leagues. These criteria are merely icing on the cake. Kids in sports just want to have a good time, be with their pals, compete, learn how to play the sport, and get as hot, sweaty, and filthy as possible.

Along the same lines, adults far too often confuse winning with having fun because winning is the measure of success in adult lives. For kids, success in sports mostly means having fun. In fact, winning at all costs usually gets in the way of having fun; the game becomes too serious. A good coach will know how to motivate his athletes to do their best while giving them the chance to enjoy themselves as much as possible. At the Sports Medicine Clinic at Children's Hospital I see the products of well-organized sports programs every day: happy, healthy, confident youngsters with a glint in their eye that tells me they're hooked on sports for life. If there's one memory that adults should have when looking back on their childhood sports, it's an overwhelming sense of fun. That virtually guarantees a lifetime interest in sports and fitness.

Organized sports have the potential to give children all the rewards described above. I'm sometimes in awe of the positive impact sports can have, especially on children with chronic illness or handicaps. As we'll see in later chapters, sports and fitness activities are emerging as an important rehabilitative tool for conditions ranging from asthma to multiple sclerosis.

The Need for Leadership

Unfortunately, our sports programs turn out so many well-adjusted child athletes *in spite of* the way they are run, not because of it. The organization of children's sports programs in this country is astoundingly haphazard. America simply hasn't responded adequately to the enormous changes involved in moving from unstructured activity to planned programs. You might argue that our "nonsystem" is working quite well — "If it ain't broke, don't fix it." But much of the evidence suggests that if our system ain't completely broke, it could certainly use some fixing. Otherwise, how do you explain the shocking fact that over 70 percent of our kids drop out of organized sports before the age of fifteen? How do you explain children's plunging fitness levels? How do you explain the new phenomenon of debilitating overuse injuries? How do you explain that organized sports have a 20 percent reinjury rate attributable to inadequate rehabilitation? These facts tell me that while there is great potential in our children's sports programs, the present situation is far from perfect.

I'm especially concerned about the quality of adult leadership, especially in coaching. Think about it: we allow coaches to make our children run laps, lift weights, perform strenuous athletic tasks, and engage in many other potentially injurious activities. Yet in most cases we don't require volunteer coaches to have any training in injury prevention, techniques for safe training and playing, or basic first aid. This highly unsatisfactory situation

Whose Hands Are You Putting Your Child In?

●

Coaches of youth sports:

- Are volunteers.
- Are role models.
- Should have some training in conditioning, exercise physiology, or psychology.
- Should be certified in first aid and CPR.
- Should have first aid supplies available on the field.
- Should have an emergency plan in the event a child is injured.
- Should be certified by the National Youth Sports Coaches Association, the American Coaching Effectiveness Program, or the Program for Athletic Coaches Education.
- May be putting children's health at risk if they are not certified.

exists partly because the demand for youth sports coaches far exceeds the supply, and most programs are reluctant to impose even minimum standards. As one sports organizer said, "Beggars can't be choosers." Although the vast majority of volunteer coaches are well meaning and committed, most simply do not have the training they should have, even though such training is available from numerous organizations.*

---

*The following organizations provide excellent coaching courses: the American Coaching Effectiveness Program (ACEP), the National Youth Sports Coaches' Association (see the Appendix under "Health, Fitness, and Safety," for addresses and phone numbers), and the Program for Athletic Coaches' Education (PACE), 213 I. M. Sports Circle, Michigan State University, East Lansing, MI 48824. Phone (517) 353-6689. For more information on youth sports certification programs,

Although I sometimes tire of comparisons between the health care system in the United States and that in Canada — a nation with a much smaller and more homogeneous population — I'm afraid our neighbors to the north are ahead of us when it comes to youth sports. All Canadian youth sports coaches must be certified by examination. Australia and New Zealand are following suit and will have mandatory certification by 1992.

I am convinced that certification of coaches will eventually come to this country, probably by the year 2000. When it does, it will be a win, win, win situation. Our coaches will win: they'll be better trained and therefore more knowledgeable in sports technique, health fitness principles, and injury prevention. Parents will win: they'll know that their children are being instructed by qualified personnel. And of course, the biggest winners will be our kids: they'll be better trained, less likely to be injured, and more qualified to participate in sports and health fitness activities throughout life.

Without training, most volunteer coaches wind up running their programs as they think a professional coach would. Too often, their criterion for success is the team's win-loss record, not whether the kids are having fun. These coaches subscribe to Vince Lombardi's credo: "Winning isn't everything; it's the only thing." I prefer the motto of the American Coaching Effectiveness Program: "Athletes first, winning second."

Therefore, while I sing the praises of organized sports for children, it troubles me greatly that too many American children are denied the very rewards these programs should provide. I'm also very concerned about the enormous numbers of kids who leave sports programs because they're cut from the team, injured, or just fed up with the overcompetitiveness. Indeed, for every potential reward sports offers, there's also the potential for a negative experience.

---

contact the National Youth Sports Foundation, 10 Meredith Circle, Needham, MA 02192. Phone (617) 449-2499.

Here's what two people arguing the pros and cons of organized sports might sound like:

Pro: Organized sports are good for kids' health because they get systematic exercise in a psychologically sound environment.

Con: Kids stand around in organized sports too much to get fit, and competition increases the risk of psychological harm.

Pro: Organized sports are safer than free play and sandlot sports.

Con: There's no proof that organized sports are safer. In fact, kids never suffered overuse injuries until organized sports came along.

Pro: Difficult sports skills and playing techniques can be learned only in a supervised sports environment, with proper coaching and officiating.

Con: Team play spawns conformity rather than individuality, and acceptance rather than innovation.

Pro: Leagues, team rankings, and tournaments make it more fun for the kids.

Con: There's no evidence that organized competition is any more enjoyable.

The simple fact is that organized sports can be either good or bad. Whether your youngster has a safe and successful experience depends almost entirely on the quality of the program he is enrolled in. If the quality of adult supervision is high, our kids can achieve all the rewards that sports have to offer.

Parents, Get Involved

No longer can we just shoo our kids out the door and say, "Go for it." Parents must act as ombudsmen for their children in the sports arena. The *American Heritage Dictionary* defines an ombudsman as "one that investigates complaints . . . and assists in achieving fair settlements." Parents act as ombudsmen in many areas of their children's lives, but involving yourself in your youngster's sports program is especially critical. There is the potential for physical and psychological harm resulting from a negative experience in sports.

Special attention must be paid to safety. Children in organized sports programs shouldn't be pushed so hard that they sustain acute or overuse injuries. When injuries occur, as they inevitably do at some point, they shouldn't be dismissed as "just part of the game." Sending a child back into action before an injury has healed can be disastrous. Above all, parents must try to make sure that the coaches in charge are qualified. If there is no certification program available in your community, then push for such a program. To see if your community sports programs meet accepted minimum safety standards, answer the questions in the safety quiz on page 36. If you answer no to any of these questions, you should demand or make changes in your community sports programs.

Another area where parents must act as ombudsmen for their children is in school sports and fitness programs. Most American schools provide too little exercise for children and gear their sports programs to an elite few. The implications of this are especially upsetting if we take into consideration children's declining opportunities for free play. Chapter 3 discusses how parents can persuade schools to perform the job they are entrusted to do in sports and fitness — with a couple of new twists.

It's essential to remember that community and school programs are inherently reactive. In other words, don't expect the quality of programs to improve without some prodding from the community. The question is whether those in the community will do the prodding. Armed with the information and advice in this book, I hope you will feel better qualified to act as an ombudsman for your child.

How Safe Are Children's Sports in Your Community?

•

1. Are all the coaches in your community — those involved in after-school sports as well as volunteers who run youth leagues — certified in first aid and CPR?

2. Are the coaches certified by the National Youth Sports Coaches Association, the American Coaching Effectiveness Program, or the Program for Athletic Coaches Education?

3. Does the coach have a written emergency plan in case of an accident, and has it been rehearsed?

4. Is there a first aid box and ice *on site* at all practices and games?

5. Does the coach have the youngsters do warm-ups, stretching, and cool-down exercises?

6. Does your school system have a sports injury prevention course as part of the health education program?

7. Are pre-sports physicals required?

8. Does the coach hand out a conditioning program before the children go out for a team so they know what will be expected of them physically?

Choosing a Sport

If you've decided that you want your child to play sports — and I hope you have — then the next important question to answer is "Which sport?" Parents often ask me if there's a perfect sport for their child. If I haven't met the youngster, my answer is always the same: "Perfect for what?" There's no one sport that does it all — builds fitness, develops motor coordination, encourages socialization with other kids, and has all the other desirable benefits of sports. For example, baseball helps develop hand-eye coordination, but doesn't do much for kids' heart-lung endurance; long-distance running is a wonderful fitness builder, but it involves little teamwork and doesn't develop motor skills.

Therefore, a more appropriate question than "Which sport?" is "Which sports?" I'm strongly in favor of youngsters playing as many sports as they can in the course of a year, providing they have good adult supervision. Playing several sports keeps kids busy and fit and allows them to develop several sports skills, which gives them options for staying fit in later life. They will also be exposed to different social situations and different groups of children.

You may be surprised to learn that the broad range of skills and fitness a child develops by playing several sports helps prevent injuries such as sprains, strains, and fractures. Sprained ankles typically occur when athletes are inexperienced in the sport or when they're tired. And overuse injuries, such as Little League elbow, shin splints, and swimmer's shoulder, are seen far more often in children who specialize in one or perhaps two sports. Lower injury rates make a strong case in favor of children pursuing diversity in sports. (Acute and overuse injuries are discussed in greater depth in Chapters 4 and 5.)

Helping your youngster select a sport is not an exact science. I wish I had a mathematical formula I could punch into a computer to find out whether a child will get hooked on softball, soccer, or gymnastics! Unfortunately, it's not that easy. But there *is* one rule you should adhere to: the choice should belong to your child. Too often, I've seen moms and dads trying to channel their kids into the sports they enjoyed or excelled in when they were younger. And some parents even push children into certain sports to improve the family's standing in the community. These folks tell me it's "for their own good" that they're waking their son or daughter every morning at six for swimming practice or driving them to tennis practice every day after school, when it's clear to me the parents are trying to achieve success vicariously through their offspring.

It's natural to want your child to succeed. What parent wouldn't want to be sitting in the front row at Wimbledon while their daughter is serving in the final for game, set, and match? But parents must resist the temptation to push their children too hard into one sport. You're probably deluding yourself if you have dreams of turning your youngster into a professional athlete. Only one in about 100,000 child athletes will make the pros. That still doesn't deter the parents who are determined to make sports stars out of their kids. These parents often justify their behavior by citing the case of Jimmy Connors. Gloria Connors had young Jimmy playing with a sawed-off racket at age two, all the while screaming at him, "Get those tiger juices going!" But for every Jimmy Connors, there are thousands and thousands of kids with burned-out minds and blown-out elbows sustained while trying to achieve someone else's goals. Do you remember Tracy Austin, the promising young tennis player who reached the Wimbledon finals in her mid-teens? It's no surprise you haven't heard her name recently: due to a chronic overuse injury, she could barely lift her right arm above her shoulder, let alone serve a tennis ball.

Remember, your child may not be interested in the sport you've picked for her. Your love of football or gymnastics isn't hereditary. Children who are pushed too hard into a sport usually find it difficult to live up to their parents' expectations. They're consistently being set up for failure. As we'll see in the chapter on psychological injuries in sports, competitive stress is one of the main reasons kids drop out of sports. Competitive stress can take away all the pleasure of the experience and can make it difficult for the child to perform well, unlike adults, who may benefit from tension.

When children aren't enjoying a sport picked out by their parents, they seldom come right out and say so. Fearful of letting their parents down, many kids grin and bear it until their parents no longer exert the same influence over them, and then they drop the sport like a hot potato, along with all interest in sports and fitness activities. An even more insidious problem is that children who do not enjoy the sport they are playing tend to sustain real or psychosomatic injuries in order to get out of it. In their minds this is an honorable way of escaping without disappointing their parents. Some signs that your youngster may not be coping well with the stresses of a sport are hyperactivity coupled with depression, disrupted sleep, rashes, nausea, headaches, muscle stiffness, lethargy, sadness, frequent unexplained illness, and loss of interest in training and competing. (See Chapter 6 for more on psychological injuries.)

Your children's desires should be uppermost, and your responsibility is to support their choice of a sport. Let your youngsters have plenty of alternatives so that they can find an enjoyable activity. A good way to help them choose is to take them to watch some community sports to see which ones capture their fancy. Some youngsters are turned off by collision sports like football and ice hockey, but fascinated by gymnastics or swimming, and vice versa.

Often kids decide to go out for a particular sport because all their pals are doing it. There's nothing wrong with that, and there's much to be said for your child feeling at ease with several of the other players in the sports program. But if it becomes clear that your child really doesn't like the sport, even with friends in the program, give her the chance to discontinue the sport and find one that is enjoyable. But first, make sure it's the sport that's the problem, not the program. Soccer is a terrific sport for most kids, but if the coach is a slave driver, the balls too old and heavy, or the goalkeeper a bully who keeps picking on your eight-year-old, then it's probably not the right program. But he might have a wonderful time in the soccer program in the next community.

Picking a suitable sport is easier if you take into account your child's strengths and weaknesses. If children are good at something, chances are they will enjoy it. Children who mature early tend to be good at most sports due to their large size and well-developed motor skills. These youngsters rarely have trouble finding a sport they enjoy. They're the ones who can throw a baseball hardest and kick a soccer ball farthest. It's the late bloomers who may find it difficult to find a suitable sport at this early stage. Often they're smaller than their peers and lacking in motor skills. Here's where parents must go all out to find an activity that suits this child.

In recent years the scope of children's sports has widened tremendously from the narrow focus on "traditional" team sports. Parents must rid themselves of the preconception that sports are just football, baseball, basketball, and hockey. There's a sport for every child if you look hard enough. If your child doesn't enjoy team sports or finds it difficult to achieve success in these areas, encourage him to choose one that doesn't require as much power, speed, agility, and balance. Jogging, cycling, canoeing, and backpacking, unlike many team sports, have the advantage of being accessible and playable for a lifetime. Children should be strongly encouraged to participate in at least one of these lifetime, or "carryover" sports, which are essential for health and fitness all through our lives.

Some parents are adamantly opposed to their children participating in a collision sport like football or hockey because of the physical contact inherent in these sports. It's worth clearing up one misconception for the record: although football and hockey certainly have their share of collision-related injuries, the supposedly safe sports, such as jogging, swimming, and aerobic dance, have their own injury problems — overuse injuries in particular. All sports carry the risk of injury. Our role as adults is to minimize the potential for injury.

Certain medical conditions may keep your child from participating in some sports. Physicians using the guidelines on disqualifying conditions published by the American Academy of Pediatrics (see Chapter 7) usually recommend that children with a single kidney shouldn't play collision or contact sports. Loose-jointed children are particularly susceptible to injuries in contact sports and should be steered toward noncontact sports such as track and field or rowing. The pre-sports physical exam should alert the physician to such conditions. In the case of kids with tight or weak muscles, the experienced sports physician will prescribe exercises to remedy these problems before the season begins. For more on the pre-sports physical, an important component of preventive sports medicine, refer to Chapter 7.

Your child's personality has a great deal to do with the choice of a sport. You are the person who knows your child best, so you are the one most qualified to judge which ones will suit her best. Extroverted, gregarious kids aren't likely to pick swimming or distance running; they're better suited to team sports like soccer or football. By the same token, shy and withdrawn youngsters often feel uncomfortable with the boisterous, chummy atmosphere of team sports. Parents often pressure shy children to join a team sport to "bring them out of their shells." This rarely seems to work. Quieter children usually don't become "wild and crazy guys" when they're thrust into that kind of environment. And, there's nothing wrong with not being on a team. Just as some people can't stand the loneliness of the long-distance runner, many others aren't interested in the camaraderie of team sports. What counts is whether your child enjoys the sport. If a child can develop self-esteem through a sport, no matter what it is, she will develop into a more confident, healthy, self-assured young person.

What follows is a rundown of the most popular youth sports divided by season. I recommend your child play at least two sports, including one or more lifetime sports. Each sport is rated for its lifetime, fitness, and injury potentials.

Fall: Cross-Country Running, Soccer, Football, Field Hockey

Cross-country running is one of the simplest sports to learn. Almost any child who adopts a slow, progressive training regimen can learn to enjoy running and also become very fit in the process. However, young runners and their coaches and parents tend to underestimate the potential for injury in this sport. I see an enormous number of knee and foot injuries in young runners caused by an overly rapid progression of training.

Lifetime potential: very high
Fitness potential: very high
   Heart-lung benefits: very high
   Strength and flexibility benefits: low
   Body composition benefits: very high
Trauma injury potential: low
Overuse injury potential: high

Soccer is an excellent sport for children. They can start playing at an early age and learn skills, conditioning, and coordination. It is a sport that can be played in later life. The standard of coaching in the United States is uneven but is improving.

Lifetime potential: high
Fitness potential
   Heart-lung benefits: very high
   Strength and flexibility benefits: moderate
   Body composition benefits: very high
Trauma injury potential: moderate
Overuse injury potential: moderate

Football teaches teamwork and specific skills related to running or impact games. The youngster who isn't particularly coordinated or good at running and endurance may still be able to play certain positions, such as line. Football provides little in the way of either a heart-lung workout or strength and flexibility training. Below the age of fourteen, this sport is very safe, with injury rates similar to those in soccer. Injury rates soar after this age, however. Participation in football can be expensive because a wide range of equipment is needed. And the equipment must be carefully maintained and repaired to minimize the potential for injury. Football is not a lifetime sport.

Lifetime potential: low
Fitness potential
   Heart-lung benefits: low
   Strength and flexibility benefits: moderate
   Body composition benefits: low
Trauma injury potential: high
Overuse injury potential: moderate

Field hockey is an open, running sport that is excellent for building heart-lung endurance. There is a very real potential for injuries, especially sprains, of the foot and ankle, and there is always the chance of being hit by a hockey stick.

Lifetime potential: low
Fitness potential
   Heart-lung benefits: very high
   Strength and flexibility benefits: moderate
   Body composition benefits: very high
Trauma injury potential: moderate
Overuse injury potential: low

Winter: Gymnastics, Basketball, Volleyball, Swimming, Wrestling, Ice Hockey, Squash, Cross-Country Skiing

Gymnastics is an excellent sport for developing strength, coordination, and flexibility. Community-based programs are widespread, and the youngster who shows proficiency in balance and tumbling can progress quickly at this level. However, the sport has several inherent risks, including the danger of catastrophic injury to the head and neck, though this risk has been reduced dramatically by controlling the use of trampolines. There is also the potential for both acute and overuse injuries. Patterns of overuse injuries to growth plates in the wrists are being detected in young female gymnasts. In fact, gymnastics is sometimes referred to as the "football of noncontact sports" because of the potential for knee, back, and arm injuries.

Lifetime potential: low
Fitness potential
  Heart-lung benefits: low
  Strength and flexibility benefits: very high
  Body composition benefits: moderate
Trauma injury potential: high
Overuse injury potential: high

Basketball is widely available and provides both excellent coordination development and a good heart-lung workout. It can also be played into middle age, thanks to the existence of well-organized leagues. Injuries to the feet, ankles, and knees are common, especially if care isn't taken to wear properly fitted shoes. Fortunately, tremendous advances in basketball shoe designs have reduced these injuries.

Lifetime potential: high
Fitness potential

  Heart-lung benefits: very high
  Strength and flexibility benefits: moderate
  Body composition benefits: very high
 Trauma injury potential: moderate
 Overuse injury potential: moderate

Volleyball is a fast-moving, highly enjoyable sport that helps develop hand-eye coordination. It is a lifetime sport that can be played recreationally even by the elderly. However, volleyball provides little in the way of conditioning.

Lifetime potential: very high
Fitness potential
  Heart-lung benefits: low
  Strength and flexibility benefits: moderate
  Body composition benefits: low
Trauma injury potential: moderate
Overuse injury potential: low

Swimming is an excellent sport that builds all three components of fitness. However, organized swimming now puts great emphasis on longer training distances. Children on teams are often encouraged by parents and coaches to focus on swimming at the expense of all other sports. As a result, ten- and eleven-year-olds, who may be swimming up to 10,000 yards a day, are subject to overuse injuries, particularly of the shoulder and knee.

Lifetime potential: very high
Fitness potential
  Heart-lung benefits: very high
  Strength and flexibility benefits: high
  Body composition benefits: very high
Trauma injury potential: low
Overuse injury potential: moderate

Wrestling is a good sport for a youngster who enjoys contact sports but isn't big enough to participate in basketball, football, or ice hockey. The different weight classes and divisions allow kids to compete with others of their size. A chronic problem in youth wrestling is inappropriate weight loss. Boys try to make lower weight classes by starving themselves of food and water, which can be very dangerous for their growth, particularly if they go below safe percentages of fat in body composition. Because wrestling is a contact sport, there is a very real potential for injuries, particularly to the knees.

Lifetime potential: low
Fitness potential
   Heart-lung benefits: moderate
   Strength and flexibility benefits: high
   Body composition benefits: moderate
Trauma injury potential: high
Overuse injury potential: low

Ice hockey is a breathtakingly fast team sport that enables child athletes to develop skating skills, balance, and coordination. It is also good for heart-lung conditioning. In some parts of the country there are opportunities for lifetime participation in no-check leagues. However, youth ice hockey has shown a disturbing trend toward winning at all costs. This drives up injury rates and cuts down on heart-lung conditioning because of the frequency of substitutions. In grade school hockey injury rates are very low because checking isn't allowed.

Lifetime potential: moderate
Fitness potential
   Heart-lung benefits: high
   Strength and flexibility benefits: moderate
   Body composition benefits: high

Trauma injury potential: high
Overuse injury potential: moderate

Squash and *racquetball* are highly skilled indoor racket sports that can help children develop hand-eye coordination and balance. Played well, they provide a vigorous heart-lung workout. Both sports can be played throughout life, and competition is widespread for people in their fifties, sixties, and even seventies. Unfortunately, squash courts are in limited supply and are concentrated in the northeast. Also, because squash requires a great deal of skill, the early stages of learning the sport can be frustrating for children. Racquetball is easier to learn and there are more courts. In both sports safety goggles must be worn to prevent eye injuries.

Lifetime potential: very high
Fitness potential
   Heart-lung benefits: high
   Strength and flexibility benefits: moderate
   Body composition benefits: very high
Trauma injury potential: moderate
Overuse injury potential: moderate

Cross-country skiing has the advantage of not being dependent on formal ski sites. It provides an excellent heart-lung workout and also builds muscles in arms, shoulders, and legs. It's a near-perfect form of exercise because it involves both athletic skill and fitness. However, there is a real potential for overuse injuries. When cross-country skiing is done on open and rolling terrain as well as on hill tracks, overuse knee injuries are common. The sport is not available in all regions of the country.

Lifetime potential: very high
Fitness potential

Heart-lung benefits: very high
Strength and flexibility benefits: very high
Body composition benefits: very high
Trauma injury potential: low
Overuse injury potential: moderate

Spring: Baseball/Softball, Track and Field, Lacrosse, Tennis

Baseball and *softball* are skilled games that help kids develop co-ordination and balance. Both are widely available, and qualified coaches are abundant. These sports are highly competitive and there may be excessive emphasis on winning and pressure on youngsters to devote all their time, energy, and emotional attention to the sport. Often these intense pressures can result in injuries.

Lifetime potential: moderate
Fitness potential
    Heart-lung benefits: low
    Strength and flexibility benefits: moderate
    Body composition benefits: low
Trauma injury potential: moderate
Overuse injury potential: high

Track and field, if properly coached, can improve a youngster's heart-lung endurance and power. The sport includes such a variety of running, jumping, and throwing events that a reasonably adept child will almost always find a niche in which to develop talent. However, the quality of coaching is highly variable, and track is not available in all regions. In certain events, such as the pole vault and high jump, there is the potential for catastrophic injury, and overuse injuries are common in the throwing events.

Lifetime potential: low
Fitness potential
   Heart-lung benefits: moderate
   Strength and flexibility benefits: moderate
   Body composition benefits: moderate
Trauma injury potential: moderate
Overuse injury potential: moderate

Lacrosse is a wonderful skill-oriented sport that develops both hand-eye coordination and heart-lung endurance. Injury levels are well below those in football and can be kept to a minimum if the equipment is used and maintained properly. Well-fitted helmets and face masks are necessary to prevent eye and face injuries.

   Lifetime potential: low
   Fitness potential
      Heart-lung benefits: very high
      Strength and flexibility benefits: moderate
      Body composition benefits: very high
   Trauma injury potential: moderate
   Overuse injury potential: moderate

Tennis is a skill-oriented sport that teaches children hand-eye coordination and, when played well, provides a good heart-lung workout. An early introduction to tennis will enable children to play competitively as well as recreationally. Tennis is one of the most highly pressured, regimented sports for kids in this country today. A child who shows early promise is often encouraged to pursue this sport to the exclusion of other activities. There is a strong emphasis on special schools and camps to maximize potential. As a result, burnout, both physical (Tracy Austin) and mental (Andrea Jaeger), is not uncommon.

Lifetime potential: very high
Fitness potential
   Heart-lung benefits: high
   Strength and flexibility benefits: moderate
   Body composition benefits: moderate
Trauma injury potential: low
Overuse injury potential: moderate

Guidelines for Young Athletes and Their Parents

Because of problems that have been seen in organized children's sports in recent years, experts in the field have drawn up several lists of guidelines. Probably the best known is the "Bill of Rights for Young Athletes," written by two prominent youth sports psychologists, Rainer Martens and Vern Seefeldt. Another is the "Code of Ethics for Parents," by Robert J. Rotella and Linda K. Bunker, which appeared in their book *Parenting Your Superstar.* I think both of these sets of guidelines should be made available to all parents and coaches. I would like to see them blown up giant size and put on a billboard that looms above every baseball diamond, gymnasium, football field, and wherever else sports are played.

Bill of Rights for Young Athletes
- The right to participate in sports
- The right to participate at a level commensurate with each child's developmental level
- The right to have qualified adult leadership

- The right to participate in safe and healthy environments
- The right to share in the leadership and decision-making of their sport
- The right to play as a child and not as an adult
- The right to proper preparation for participation in sports
- The right to an equal opportunity to strive for success
- The right to be treated with dignity
- The right to have fun in sports

Code of Ethics for Parents
- I will help my child learn to enjoy sports and develop the skills that he or she is capable of performing.
- I will learn the strengths and weaknesses of my child so that I may place the young athlete in situations where he or she has a maximum opportunity for success.
- I will become thoroughly familiar with the techniques and rules of the sport my child chooses.
- I will do my best to learn the fundamental teaching skills and strategies related to my child's sport.
- I will practice and help my child so that he or she will have an opportunity for skill improvement through active participation.
- I will communicate with my child the rights and responsibilities of others who are involved in sport.
- I will protect the health and safety of my child by insisting that all of the activities under my control are conducted in accord with his or her psychological and physiological welfare.
- I will treat each player, opposing coach, official, parent, and administrator with respect and dignity.
- I will uphold the authority of officials and coaches who are working with my child. I will assist them when possible and use good judgment if I disagree with them.
- I will become familiar with the objectives of the sports programs with which my child is affiliated.

- I will strive to help select activities that uphold our family values.
- I will help my child develop good sportsmanship and a desire to strive for success.

So to answer your question, "Should my child play sports?" I'd look you square in the eye and draw from my twenty years of experience in pediatric and adolescent sports medicine and give you a definitive "Yes . . . and no." What I mean is this: "Absolutely not" if you're going to force your youngster into a program against her will, or enter her willy-nilly into any program that happens to be convenient. "Definitely yes" if you're willing to recognize that the demands of sports have changed and that you must respond to this change if your child is to get the most out of the program.

3

• • • • •

Health Fitness for
Children's Sports . . . and Life!

Recently I reread a favorite short story about a future society in which humans have evolved into quivering, blubbery mounds of translucent flesh. They live in tiny cubicles deep in the earth, communicating and entertaining themselves without having to move, using telephones and televisions. Sounds totally absurd, doesn't it? But think: we're closer to this lifestyle than to that of our great-grandparents. Compared to our ancestors, we're leading exceedingly sedentary lives. Thank goodness we began to recognize this harmful trend about twenty years ago, and so the fitness boom was born. Although Americans still need to improve their health fitness levels, at least we've faced up to the need for physical activity in our lives. In many cases we've acted on this knowledge. But before we strain a muscle patting ourselves on the back, just remember that while many adults have jogged, biked, or "aerobicized" their way to better health fitness, we've left behind a very significant group: our children.

Despite the explosion in organized children's sports, children's health fitness levels have never been lower. Gortmaker, Dietz, and colleagues analyzed nationally representative data and found that obesity in adolescents increased 39 percent between the beginning of the 1960s and the start of the 1980s. Over half of a group of 360 kids recently tested couldn't perform *one* measly chin-up, and a third of that group couldn't do more than ten minutes of moderate exercise. In a study of school-age children in Michigan, researchers discovered that 41 percent had high cholesterol, 28 percent had high triglycerides, and 28 percent had high blood pressure, all of which are risk factors for heart disease. A very recent study of four million youngsters revealed that a full *two thirds* were below the basic level of health fitness when they were asked to jog, do sit-ups, and do a touch-your-toes test.

What Is Health Fitness?

You may not have heard this term before you picked up this book. As I have explained, health fitness includes a strong heart and lungs (cardiovascular fitness), strength and flexibility (musculoskeletal fitness), and an appropriate muscle-fat ratio (nutritional fitness).

The problem is, people often assume that organized sports naturally build health fitness. That's simply not true, which is part of the reason that the growth in organized sports has been paralleled by a decline in children's fitness levels. There is some overlap — health fitness does improve performance in certain sports, and some sports do enhance areas of health fitness — but traditional youth sports are generally geared toward performing skills like hitting a ball or breaking through a tackle, not developing endurance, strength, and flexibility. To illustrate the confusion that exists, remember that until very recently, fitness testing in schools measured attributes like speed, power, and agility. These are nice to have, but they contribute almost nothing to our health.

In part because of the confusion surrounding these concepts, our children's fitness levels have plunged to the levels we see today. Traditional health fitness-building activities like free play and sandlot sports have been replaced by organized sports, which, it was assumed, would do the same job. However, although sports such as baseball and football may be terrific fun and a valuable means of socialization for our kids, they are often not nearly as effective as free play was in building health fitness. To put it bluntly, Little League baseball and Pop Warner football aren't as health-building as a vigorous game of tag.

Unfortunately, our misconceptions about what constitutes fitness often lead us to believe that when our kids are involved in traditional organized sports they're fulfilling their health fitness requirements. Too often they're not. It's essential to recognize the difference between sports-specific skills and health fitness, and to encourage our children to participate in activities that will develop both.

The Decline of Health Fitness

It is unfair to blame children's declining health fitness entirely on the rise of organized sports. The fact is that outside of whatever sports they play, if any, children today are leading extremely sedentary lives. They have been shackled to the twin pillars of late twentieth-century America: television and the automobile. Instead of walking to and from school or to a friend's house as they did a generation ago, kids are shuttled about in the schoolbus or the family station wagon. Sandlot sports have been replaced by cartoons and video games. Say what you will about "interactive" computer games for kids, to me they're just plain "*in*active."

Parents' concerns for their children's safety away from home lead to more dependence on these modern amenities. Given the highly publicized horror stories of child abduction that appear in our newspapers and on TV every day, it's not surprising that many adults, especially working parents, who are away from home all day, instruct their "latchkey kids" to "go home, lock the door, and watch television till I get home."

The loss of open space and vacant lots in many cities and suburbs has also put an end to traditional health fitness-enhancing activities ranging from tag to pick-up basketball. In the inner cities many of the remaining play areas have been overrun by drug dealers and other undesirable elements. No wonder concerned city parents tell their kids to stay home and watch TV when too many of the youngsters at the local playground end up shooting drugs instead of baskets.

Watching TV for hours on end not only cuts down on physical activity but also increases "nutritional delinquency" because kids love to snack on foods high in fat and sodium while they watch. In a study of children's TV viewing habits in relation to obesity, it was revealed that in adolescents aged twelve to seventeen, obesity increased 2 percent for each hour of TV watched. Heavily sugared, salted, and otherwise modified foods now comprise over 55 percent of the American family's food intake. Changes in Americans' eating habits over the last couple of generations have added nutritional unfitness to the list of children's health fitness woes.

As if all this weren't bad enough, federal cutbacks in education have led to the slashing of budgets for physical education in school. Compared to the three R's, the assumption goes, physical education is "frivolous." Unbelievably, only about one third of American high schools provide their students with the daily p.e. activity recommended by the U.S. Department of Health and Human Services for basic health fitness.

Benefits of Health Fitness

So what if children's health fitness levels are plunging? The answer to this question isn't as simple as it might appear. We know

The Benefits of Health Fitness

●

Vigorous physical activity:

- Increases the number and size of blood vessels in the heart and the muscles, resulting in better and more efficient circulation.

- Increases the elasticity of blood vessels, lessening the likelihood of breakage under pressure.

- Increases the efficiency of exercising muscles, enabling the muscles and blood to better carry and utilize oxygen.

- Increases the efficiency of the heart, making it a better pump.

- Increases tolerance to stress, reducing the negative effects of the stress/pressure syndrome.

- Decreases cholesterol and triglycerides, lessening the chances of arterial deposits.

- Lowers high blood pressure, reducing the risk of heart attack and stroke.

Adapted from D. F. Haydon, "The Family and Health/Fitness," *Health Values* 11(2):36–39 (1987).

that it's better to be fit than unfit and that fitness begets healthiness, but many Americans would be hard pressed to explain why. The benefits of health fitness are many and varied, especially for sports-active children (see the box above).

Health fitness beginning in childhood helps avert chronic illnesses in later life. There are now forty years' worth of studies clearly linking heart-lung endurance (cardiovascular fitness) with a reduced incidence of, and death rate from, stroke and heart disease. Exercise also combats heart disease by lowering cholesterol levels, raising HDL ("good" cholesterol), and stabilizing blood pressure at desirable levels. Strength and flexibility (musculoskeletal fitness) are essential for preventing lower back pain. The enormous increase in back pain complaints in this country — now the second leading cause, after the common cold, of lost work days — is attributed to Americans' increased sedentarism. By increasing the density of bone minerals, exercise has also been shown to help young women avoid osteoporosis in later life; this is important for men too. Keeping levels of body fat low (nutritional fitness) is important for minimizing the risk of heart disease, hypertension, diabetes, and even certain types of cancers.

Remember also that exercise is essential to normal growth. Your child's heart, lungs, muscles, and bones cannot develop without being worked, and exercise is the most effective way of working these body components. Compared to children who lead sedentary lives, active kids tend to have bigger and stronger hearts, greater muscle mass, less fatty tissue, and stronger bones.

One of the most intriguing developments in the field of sports science research has been the link established between physical fitness and psychological health. Both anxiety and depression have been treated using fitness programs. It's also well known that people who take up exercise experience an improved sense of well-being and self-esteem. Indeed, several studies have recorded improvements in children's academic performance with increased fitness activities.

Health fitness also enhances children's sports performance. The better nourished, stronger, more flexible athlete will almost always outperform an overweight, weaker, and less flexible opponent. But much more important, fitness helps prevent injuries. The child who is unfit is much more likely to be hurt. It stands to reason that the out-of-shape soccer player who is exhausted by the second quarter is likely to trip and sprain an ankle. Strong muscles and bones can help prevent common overuse injuries such as Little League elbow, swimmer's shoulder, and gymnast's back. A child who is malnourished is more likely to sustain a fatigue-related injury, while obese children are predisposed to a host of different injuries because of the strain on their bodies during strenuous exercise.

Achieving Health Fitness

All-around health fitness is rarely achieved through practicing specific team sports skills. Certain sports do promote health fitness, such as cycling, swimming, jogging, and strength training, but our culture has resisted recognizing these activities as legitimate sports for kids. We need to encourage our children to participate in these activities. Previous generations didn't have to give health fitness-building activities much thought — they were part of their daily lives. Our ancestors had no choice but to walk to work or school, carry groceries, bale hay, do chores manually rather than by machine, and eat diets high in complex carbohydrates. All this has changed, however, and instead of relying on our normal existence to build health fitness, we now have to make a conscious effort to get the exercise our bodies need for health fitness.

Cardiovascular fitness means your heart and lungs respond effectively to the oxygen demands of exercise. Aerobic exercise is the best way to condition the cardiovascular system. In fact, the word *aerobic* means "air" (not "leotard" as one of my young patients thought!). Some good aerobic activities are jogging, biking, rowing, cross-country skiing, rope skipping, and of course, aerobic dance — in other words, anything that gets your heart pounding and your lungs pumping. To improve their cardiovascular health and endurance, your children must engage in at least twenty to thirty minutes of continuous vigorous aerobic activity three or four times a week.

Musculoskeletal fitness refers to the strength and flexibility of muscles and bones, including joints, ligaments, and cartilage.

Strength and flexibility in these structures contribute to better health and efficient body function and also to safe participation in competitive sports. Strength is increased through the "overload principle": the exercise must be sufficiently intense to overload the body's structures and yet not cause them injury. Training with free weights or weight machines is the most efficient way to build strength. Until quite recently, training with weights was thought to be harmful for children. It was also believed that before puberty youngsters were unable to increase their strength with weights. Not true! Dr. Les Sewell and I surprised many of our colleagues when we produced strength increases of 12 to 15 percent in boys and girls aged nine to eleven in a recent study. Our results, since corroborated by other studies, also showed that properly performed strength training is no more dangerous for children than it is for adults. Sit-ups are an excellent way to improve abdominal strength, which is vital for preventing lower-back pain.

Flexibility allows us to move freely and easily without stiffness and reduces or prevents muscle soreness and injury from sports. Lack of flexibility due to a sedentary lifestyle, combined with poor abdominal strength, is thought to be the cause of the dramatic increase of lower-back pain in this country over the last half century. A simple stretching program is the best way to improve flexibility.

For more on strength and flexibility, see Chapter 8.

Nutritional fitness refers to the proportion of fatty tissue to lean muscle, known as body composition. Your child's body fat should be about 20 percent of his total weight. Body fat above 25 percent in boys and 32 percent in girls signifies obesity. A tremendous problem among our youth, obesity is attributable to lack of aerobic exercise as well as a diet high in fats, sugars, and modified products. In young athletes obesity may precipitate serious problems in the legs, feet, knees, and hips. The overweight child athlete is also predisposed to heat exhaustion. Metabolic diseases such as hypertension, diabetes, and heart conditions get started more easily in the overweight child. Aerobic exercise — jogging, biking, cross-country skiing, aerobic dance, or rope skipping — is the most effective way of reducing body fat, along with a balanced diet. Chapter 9 deals in depth with nutrition for the child athlete.

What Does Fitness Testing Test?

Achieving these three components of health fitness is essential if we hope to halt our children's slide into the abyss of sedentariness, where all manner of health hazards await them. We should remember that while sports-specific skills such as speed, power, and agility are mainly inherited, health fitness is available to everyone. Your child may never have the hand-eye coordination of a Babe Ruth (they say he could count the number of stitches on a baseball heading toward the plate!), but he can certainly achieve excellent health fitness. The trouble is that we still equate speed, power, and agility with fitness. This confusion explains the traditional orientation of school-based fitness tests such as the President's Challenge, which includes a sprint; a hop, skip, and jump; a vertical jump; and a spin and turn. These movements measure congenital motor skills, not health fitness.

Another problem is that these tests tend to reward only a small percentage of the motor-skilled youngsters who are tested. The President's Challenge still recognizes only the top fifteenth percentile. Those kids who don't make that percentile are deemed more "unfit" than the elite group, when in fact, their health fitness isn't even being measured! Studies have shown that many of those children think of themselves as "naturally unfit" and drop out of sports and fitness activities forever.

Now, I'm happy to say, the approach to fitness testing in the schools is being revised. Organizations such as the American Health and Fitness Foundation and the American Alliance for Health, Physical Education, Recreation, and Dance (see the Appendix for more information) have come up with excellent programs that measure health fitness components. Even the redoubtable President's Council on Fitness has altered the President's Challenge to include more health fitness tests. Heart-lung endurance is measured with a timed jog; strength is measured by counting the number of sit-ups performed in a limited time; flexibility is measured with a touch-your-toes test; and body composition is measured using skin calipers. All of these new fitness tests are geared toward rewarding everyone who tries and not iust the kids who perform the best.

Changing Our Approaches to Sports
and Health Fitness

The new emphasis on health fitness in school testing should provide an impetus for creating new attitudes toward fitness in our society. If we are to reverse the declining levels in children's health fitness, it is essential that we radically change our approaches to fitness and sports in three areas: at home, in the schools, and in the community.

In the Home . . .

The last half century has ushered in immense changes for the American family. Sociologists tell us that as families have struggled to adapt to new living patterns — divorce, separation, working mothers, and single parents are now commonplace —

Health Fitness Profile of the American Family

●

Children

- 50 percent don't get enough exercise to develop healthy cardiorespiratory systems.
- 98 percent have at least one heart disease risk factor.
- 13 percent have five or more risk factors.
- 20–30 percent are obese.
- 75 percent consume excess fat.

Adults

- 64 percent don't get enough exercise to maintain healthy cardiorespiratory systems.
- 24 percent never exercise.
- 35 percent are overweight.
- 30 percent smoke cigarettes.

Adapted from D. F. Haydon, "The Family and Health/Fitness," *Health Values* 11(2):36–39 (1987).

parental concerns about health and fitness have been put on the back burner. The health fitness profile of American families is downright frightening (see the box above).

Charity begins at home, and so should fitness. Children emulate their parents' behavior, even when they seem most rebellious. How often did we say as kids, "I'll never act like my parents when I'm grown up"? But the next thing we know we are doing just that. For better or worse, we end up imitating many of the behavior patterns of our parents, and that includes health fitness behavior.

How do you become a good health fitness role model for your

children? To begin with, the importance of fitness should be discussed within the family. Because children resist being preached to, one of the most effective ways of having your kids understand the role of fitness is to ask them what aspects of life are important to them and how they plan to achieve their goals in these areas. Chances are that many of their goals — happiness, friendship, popularity, and longevity, for example — can be achieved or enhanced through physical activity. Having your children recognize this is very important. Once they acknowledge the role of physical fitness, you can focus on the benefits described in this chapter.

However, it would be wrong to discuss only the benefits of physical activity. The problems of staying fit in our society must also be addressed, especially with the time constraints we all face. Your youngsters must learn to make time for fitness activities. If you are involved in a fitness program, you can use your experiences to describe the problems and rewards of fitness. Your children should come away from the discussion feeling that almost anyone who wants to can become fit. The ideal way to cap a talk about the benefits of fitness is for the family to engage in some physical activity together, such as taking a walk or a jog or cycling.

A positive attitude toward health fitness has to be more than symbolic. You can set simple, everyday good examples for your children to follow. Here are three: don't use the elevator — *use the stairs*. Don't use a self-propelled mower — *use a push mower*. Don't drive to the convenience store — *walk or cycle the distance*. Your kids may occasionally complain about the extra exercise — they wouldn't be kids if they didn't — but you'll be surprised at how quickly they adapt to it. Don't be surprised when they start following these everyday health fitness rules automatically and take them into adulthood.

Some exercise therapists advocate introducing good health fitness values at a very early age. Charles Kuntzelman, one of our most progressive child fitness thinkers, whose Feelin' Good program is based in Michigan, writes:

> Toddlers shouldn't be restrained in playpens; they should be given the chance to move about freely and explore. You should make a habit of turning on the stereo at home and encouraging your child to move to the music. You can encourage them by moving about a lot yourself, however silly you might feel! If mom and dad are going for a walk they should take baby along with them in a "kiddy sack" or a stroller; bikers can put the child in a back seat. That way the child is instinctively learning that physical activity is important.
>
> Birthdays are a terrific opportunity to create positive feelings about health fitness in your children. Try this: go for a family walk on the day of your child's birthday, going a bit farther each year. As your child gets older this will become a family tradition, and each mile added will make your youngster feel more mature. Birthday party activities should be active. A vigorous game of tag is infinitely preferable to "pin the tail on the donkey." Birthday presents should encourage fitness; give your children a bike, sneakers, or skis. As they get older, your youngsters will associate these important days with an important part of life: health fitness.

Recent studies have shown that parents participate with their children in strenuous physical activity only once a week on average. It's vital that you engage in health fitness activities with your children. I'm not talking here about driving them to the Little League game. What I mean is that you should choose an activity that both you and your child enjoy and do it together regularly. There are plenty of activities to choose from: walking, jogging, backpacking, and swimming are just a few. Don't forget that kids have short attention spans, and they shouldn't be restricted to just one activity, or even one at a time. If you go for a walk with your child, take along a skipping rope, a soccer ball, a kite — or all of them! — to keep your child occupied. Above all, the activity should be fun. Your kids won't respond to the concept of doing something just because it's good for them — they have to enjoy it.

Charles Kuntzelman is a treasure trove of interesting ideas for family fitness. He recently told me about the "mileage club" he and his wife Beth formed with their kids. The family tallied up the miles they walked every week and plotted the distance on a map. "In a few months, a small family can walk across their state," says Charlie, "while a large family — grandparents included, of course — can walk across the whole country." To make this game even more fun, the Kuntzelman family had little celebrations along the way; the kids went to see a Disney movie when they "reached" Disneyland; when they "arrived" in Mexico, the family went out for a slap-up Mexican meal. Let's take Charlie Kuntzelman's idea a step further. If you start a mileage club with your children today, by the time your grandchildren are in college your family can have walked around the world!

Not only do these activities enhance your children's fitness, they also contribute to better family relations. The barriers that naturally develop between parents and children as they mature tend to fall when you're all huffing and puffing up a hill on your bikes. There is an unmistakable feeling of togetherness when you share these memorable experiences. And when you stop, red-faced and sweating, and look at one another, sharing a smile and a gulp of ice water, you'll realize that the family ties have been drawn a little closer.

In the Schools . . .

Just as parents often assume that their children are "naturally fit," they also tend to think that all's well in the school physical education department. Nothing could be further from the truth. Most schools have abdicated their responsibility to teach physical education. Incredibly, only 36 percent of American schools provide thirty minutes of aerobic activity per day, as recommended by the U.S. Department of Health and Human Services. And many school p.e. departments that claim they meet this requirement do so only on paper. In reality, they're simply not providing children with even the minimum needed for health fitness. Many p.e. classes are too short: they last only thirty-five minutes, and when you subtract ten minutes for changing and showering, that leaves only twenty minutes or so for physical activity.

There's also the very real concern that what's going on in those classes is unsatisfactory. I've walked in on many p.e. classes where the kids are standing around far too long to get the necessary health benefits of exercise. This problem results mainly from a lack of qualified or motivated p.e. teachers. As many as *one third* of all people teaching physical education in our schools aren't certified. As for those who are certified, fitness experts are concerned that their training may not be satisfactory. It's not all the teachers' fault, however; they are often handicapped by having to teach classes too large to allow them to give sufficient attention to individual students.

Who's to blame? It's easy to point a finger at the schools and blame the educators for not doing their job. It's just as easy to blame the politicians for cutting back funding for our schools. To an extent, we'd be justified in doing that. Our teachers do need to become more concerned with teaching, and our political leaders must give them appropriate moral and financial support for this.

But really, much of the fault lies with us. Never has parent participation in PTAs and PTOs been lower, according to Donald Haydon, executive director of the American Health and Fitness Foundation. This is just one measure of parents' declining involvement in their children's education. Significantly, as fewer parents have acted as watchdogs, the quality and quantity of p.e. in our schools have decreased. Parents are the only ones who can remedy this sorry state of affairs. Remember, schools are by their very nature reactive, not pro-active, and parents have to be the catalysts for change.

The first step is to become more involved in your children's school education. Go to the school and find out what the p.e. requirements are. Ask what the goal of the p.e. department is and, most important, how the p.e. department is fulfilling that goal. If you don't like what you see and hear, try to change it. It's important to recognize that it's *your* school system — *your* tax dollars pay for it. If you don't feel that the system is for the best interests of your child, you have every right to demand change.

But what should you be demanding? Donald Haydon suggests that all schools should have the following health fitness requirements as their goal. I wholeheartedly support his guidelines.

- Physical education should be mandatory for students from kindergarten to twelfth grade *without exception.*
- The primary objective of the p.e. curriculum should be to produce physically fit children.
- The time allotment for p.e. at both the elementary and secondary level should be at least thirty minutes of aerobic activity three times a week.
- The student–teacher ratio in p.e. classes should be reduced.
- Additional degreed p.e. teachers should be placed in schools, particularly in the lower grades.

Another important change that should be made in schools' approach to health fitness is a shift away from the traditional team sports, which tend to drain the budgets of most p.e. departments. From about the fourth grade on, children are steered toward competitive team sports at the expense of movement-related activities. A limited number of students participate in team sports, while many others must do without adequate coaching or facilities. Also the skills taught in these sports have little or no relevance for later life. As a result, we have turned into a nation of dedicated spectators, a "fat 'n' happy" bunch more interested in watching sports on TV than playing them ourselves.

Here's the question you should ask about each school sport: Can my child use this skill when he or she is forty, fifty, or seventy? The answer is usually no. I'm not saying that organized team sports should be dropped. That would be folly. My childhood, adolescence, and early adulthood were filled with football, lacrosse, and rugby, and I wouldn't have had it any other way. However, in my day the kids who didn't make one team or another had plenty of free-play opportunities and sandlot sports to help build fitness. That's no longer the case. We now rely heavily on the schools to provide our youngsters with opportunities for physical activity. Therefore school sports programs must be more *balanced*, with a greater emphasis on lifetime or carryover sports, including running, cycling, dance, swimming, and racket sports.

One of the most exciting developments in school health fitness programs has been the emergence of the so-called New Games, which have been pioneered by a small but dedicated group of exercise therapists. Their philosophy is that sports should be playful and noncompetitive. New Games require little in the way of equipment, relying instead on the training and knowledge of leaders. Because these activities are economical and can involve large numbers of kids, some schools find them an attractive alternative to existing organized sports.

New Games look totally different from anything we're used to seeing on our playing fields. First, there are likely to be no spectators, only participants. Second, the games don't require a set number of team members, so a few or many can participate. Finally, the games require a spirit of cooperation and creativity — sometimes the rules are changed in the middle of the game — that is sadly lacking in organized sports.

Characteristic of the New Games are the various Earthball activities. The Earthball is an enormous canvas ball filled with air. In tournament Earthball the ball must be pushed or otherwise propelled over a goal line. Rules may require that all participants play on their hands and knees or that the ball be propelled only by hitting it with your rear end (the "bump"). When a lot of people are playing together, the ball is in the air most of the time. In many New Games, the participants are reduced to help-less laughter for a large part of the playing time, thus achieving one of the goals of this movement — playfulness of the most childlike and enjoyable kind.

It's too early to tell whether the New Games are the wave of the future or an interesting but brief phase in the history of sports. Several factors suggest that they may be here to stay. For instance, many schools need to find cheaper alternatives to the existing team sports. Outfitting a hockey or football team and providing transportation to and from games for the team, band, and assorted coaches and managers soak up a significant portion of the school budget.

Then there is the question of participation. Team sports may involve 10 to 15 percent of a school population, with many of the others serving as spectators. The New Games have the ad-vantage that everyone can participate and benefit from the phys-ical activities. If they can teach an attitude of joyful participation at an early age and promote its continuation into adult life, the New Games will have made a strong contribution to our culture.

Physical education need not begin and end in the gym. In ad-dition to health fitness activities, another kind of curriculum can be of value to your growing child: an understanding of human physiology. Health education hasn't been held in high esteem by teachers or students. The old hygiene courses taught by the gym teacher or school nurse have in some instances been replaced by more sophisticated materials that can be taught by the regular classroom teacher. But little has been done to take advantage of kids' innate desire to be active. Their tremendous energy could be harnessed to teach them about the workings of the human body by installing a version of the cardiac physiology lab in the school. Through the simple technique of taking their pulse rate, children as young as eight have been taught to estimate their own levels of health fitness. New curricula are being developed in some schools to teach students about the relationship between exercise and nutritional fitness. Story telling, mathematical problems, art, and music can be related to motion. At the high school level, the bicycle or treadmill ergometer can be used to teach physiology in a thoroughly personal way, by letting the students assess their health fitness while learning about muscle physiology, the biochemistry of energy use, and cardiovascular function.

While a number of attempts have been made to change schools' approach to health fitness education, much more needs to be done. How can you become the all-important catalyst for change? According to Vern Seefeldt, director of the Youth Sports Institute, an organization dedicated to improving children's fitness levels, the place to begin is at the top. He suggests banding together with a group of similar-minded parents and attending the next meeting of your local school board to raise the issue of the declining quality of physical education. Three main questions must be asked: "How much p.e. are our children getting?" "Who's teaching it?" and "What goes on in the p.e. classes?" The only answers that should satisfy you are that your children are getting three forty-five-minute sessions of p.e. per week; that they are being taught by a certified p.e. teacher; and that at least thirty minutes of each p.e. class is dedicated to aerobic activity. If the answers you get don't satisfy you, ask the school board what they're going to do to improve things and when these improvements are going to be made.

Just think about it: if your kids weren't learning to read, there'd be hell to pay in the English department. Well, if they're not getting fit, something needs to be done to improve the quality of their physical education. As I write this book, plenty of reports have told us how poorly our kids are doing in school compared to their counterparts in countries like Japan, England, and Canada. So far these reports have addressed only academics and, predictably, plenty of outrage has been expressed. But nobody's addressing how badly our kids are flunking in the area of fitness, even though all the evidence suggests that their fitness levels have plunged much further than their academic performance. It's time we made p.e. a priority in our schools!

In the Community . . .

It's also important to change our approach to community health fitness. After all, an estimated 85 percent of American children participate in community sports. Health fitness at this level is really a question of facilities and leadership. Communities making decisions concerning new programs must understand the overall costs and benefits of these investments. If a choice has to be made between an ice hockey rink and a swimming pool, the health fitness benefits of the pool for the whole community may well place it above team hockey in importance. At present, decisions aren't always made on this basis. Community enthusiasm for football and hockey, often promoted through booster clubs and like-minded interests, is often the driving force in favor of building facilities for these sports. But well-reasoned arguments can be marshaled to underscore the greater health benefits of alternative facilities — which need not be expensive — such as a lighted jogging track, a cycling track, or a supervised park.

Whenever a new sports program is planned, several questions should be asked. Most parents have never attended a local recreation commission meeting. If they have, they haven't asked the following important questions:

- Does the activity contribute to the health of its users and the community in some way?
- Can the program be used by most members of the commu-

nity? — young and old, both sexes, and people with handicaps?
• Is it fun?

Community health fitness facilities need effective leadership.
Unfortunately, most *recreation* specialists or administrators don't
think enough about their role as *health* specialists. But in fact that
is what they must become if we are to make health fitness popular with our children. The business of maintaining health is not
simply a concern of the medical profession. It is a community
responsibility, which in the future is likely to belong at least in
part to recreation experts.

The methods can be simple, the facilities inexpensive. The
major need is for leadership, as numerous studies have demonstrated. As a nation, we simply don't know how to lead our citizens to better health fitness over a lifetime. The dropout rate for
most fitness programs is high. To train better leaders, our schools
will have to turn to a greater emphasis on lifetime health fitness
and physiology, so that children learn to protect their hearts and
muscles from future deterioration. Health education, currently
one of the least popular subjects in schools, should be tied closely
to the concept of fitness.

Instead of creating a new group of paramedical professionals
to carry out this mission, we need volunteer leaders at all levels,
in every school, office, and factory. Parents should set a good
fitness example for their kids at home and actively search for
health fitness activities for the family to participate in. Elementary school teachers should be trained to lead fitness programs
instead of automatically turning their students over to a physical
education teacher a few times a week. At the community level,
instruction in using fitness trails and other programs requiring
some skill should be provided by neighborhood residents who
have the appropriate training and background. All of this will
require backup, supervision, and professional training, some of

it expert in nature. But it will be far better to place this knowledge in the hands of a large number of volunteers than to reserve it for a few highly trained professionals.

It is your children and grandchildren who will ultimately benefit from these changes in approach to health fitness. It is *you* who must make it happen. Beginning at home, and spreading down your street to encompass the neighborhood, district, city or town, state, and eventually, the whole country, health fitness for our children must be given the highest priority.

4

•••••

Sports Injuries:
Just Part of the Game?

With the explosion in organized sports for children has come a dramatic increase in the number of injuries. Acute injuries, which include cuts, bruises, sprains, and fractures, are now the leading cause of hospital admissions for children and adolescents, and a frequent reason for repeated clinic visits. Many of these injuries occur in youth sports programs. The U.S. Consumer Product Safety Commission reports that four million children seek treatment for sports injuries in hospital emergency rooms every year, and it estimates that another eight million are treated for such injuries by primary care physicians. High school athletes sporting casts on an arm or leg are a common sight in most communities.

Critics tell us that organized sports are too violent or physically demanding. The price for our obsession with youth sports, paid in the hard currency of injuries, is too high, they insist, and society should allow kids to return to free play and sandlot sports.

But are organized sports themselves to blame? I think they have gotten a bad rap. Without a doubt, many of the injuries we're now seeing are caused by children's declining levels of fitness. Many observers attribute the skyrocketing incidence of sports-related injuries to the simple fact that many more kids than ever before are in sports programs. To an extent they're right. All things being equal, when you have five times as many kids playing organized football in Anytown, USA, the town's good citizens can expect five times as many sports injuries among their children.

As for whether organized sports are more dangerous than free play, there's little conclusive evidence either way. I'm not so nostalgic for the good old days that I can overlook the fact that kids also get injured in free play. During my stints in hospital emergency rooms as an intern in the sixties, I remember treating innumerable children who had fallen out of trees, biked into drains, or caught a rock in the face. Not surprisingly, it hasn't yet been determined whether your child is more likely to break an arm climbing trees or playing Pop Warner football. A few hard statistics are available. For instance, the Consumer Product Safety Commission tells us that as many children are injured every year in skateboarding accidents as on the football gridiron — about 350,000 in each category in 1985. Some supervised sports programs have far fewer serious injuries than occur in similar kinds of free play. Swimming is an obvious example: thousands of children drown every year in swimming holes and lakes, while almost no fatalities occur in organized swimming programs.

The mechanisms of acute, or trauma, injuries are identical to those of general pediatric trauma cases. In other words, the sprained ankle of a child who tumbles down the stairs at home is no different from the young soccer player's sprained ankle. And in an ideal world, these injuries would be managed identically, with the criterion for rehabilitation being complete restoration of strength, range of motion, and balance. However, I'm enormously concerned about the lack of concern shown about many children's sports injuries. Most parents are quick to haul their child to the local hospital emergency room if she falls down the stairs, but an injury on the sports field is all too often dismissed as "just part of the game." At best this laissez-faire approach delays a child's recovery, prevents her return to full function, and predisposes her to reinjury. At worst she may not be able to play the sport again and may carry long-term debilitating injuries into adulthood.

Because of the mechanism of growth, children are highly vulnerable to injuries caused by a fall, a twist, or a turn. Most growth takes place in the areas just below the bulbous points, called the epiphyses, of the upper and lower ends of the long bones. These areas are the growth plates, which are made up of bone cartilage cells that haven't yet hardened into bone. Because the growth plates are softer than the main part of the bone, they are susceptible to injury, particularly during the growth spurt of adolescence.

If a growth plate is injured, the affected bone may stop growing while the growth plate heals. Take, for instance, an injury to the growth plate of the lower thighbone (the femur) of the left leg. While that growth plate busies itself replacing damaged cells, the other leg is growing. If such an injury occurs in a twelve-year-old, the injured leg may be as much as two inches shorter if the growth fracture is left untreated. The ankle and wrist both have two main long bones, and injury to the growth plate of one may upset the delicate interaction between the two bones and cause joint dysfunction.

What may be worse than an outright fracture of the growth plate is a partial injury to it. When this happens, the bone may grow at a peculiar angle and cause serious problems. For example, I'm frequently called upon to explain to parents that the reason their child has a bowed leg or an arm that won't straighten is that he suffered a partial growth plate fracture that was ignored. Clearly, injuries in children's sports can have serious consequences, especially if untreated. It's important that parents and coaches not dismiss injuries as "just part of the game."

Part of the problem is that there is no system of effective medical care in youth sports programs. In adult sports an injured athlete presents himself to the team physician, often at the direction of the coach. If the team has an athletic trainer, he may provide an initial assessment before the athlete sees "doc." The team doctor's main job is to confirm the diagnosis, estimate the severity of the injury and, most important, determine when the athlete may return to action after appropriate treatment and rehabilitation. The doctor can rely on the cooperation of the coach and trainer in supervising the injured athlete's rehabilitation program.

Not so for the child athlete. Though one of the supposed benefits of organized sports is adult supervision and coaching in safe playing techniques, volunteer coaches simply are not trained to recognize and manage even the most straightforward of injuries or to teach safe training techniques. Little has been done to teach coaches concepts of safe training, preventive sports medicine, or first aid. Even in school physical education programs, medical supervision is fragmentary. Most states require physicians and emergency medical technicians (EMTs) to attend high school football games, but no such provision is made for junior high or grade school sports. In most cases the coaches have been drafted from the English or chemistry department, earning extra income for their coaching time.

Of this country's three and a half million coaches, from tee-ball to the pros, over 80 percent have no formal coaching training, and their knowledge of the sport they coach varies widely. On-site medical coverage may be the responsibility of the school nurse, who is often ill equipped to provide comprehensive care for injuries. Many times a parent has to drive an injured child to the family physician, pediatrician, or emergency room. This situation will probably get worse before it gets better because of funding cuts in school programs. In community sports programs, where there is no system of medical care for the kids, the situation is even more worrisome. By contrast, in college and professional sports enormous sums of money are spent to ensure full recovery of a few thousand "professional entertainers." Our kids are just as important, as far as I'm concerned, and deserve as much attention.

Preventing Sports Injuries

All sports carry some potential for injury. It's how we deal with this potential that makes the difference. Parents have three choices: you can choose to do nothing, you can yank your children from sports altogether, or you can work to minimize the risk of injury by following some fairly straightforward guidelines. I favor the last option.

The most effective way to prevent sports injuries in your children is to ensure that the program they are in is staffed by a trained coach, preferably one who has been certified by either the National Youth Sports Coaches Association or the American Coaching Effectiveness Program. At the very least, your child's coach should have training in first aid and CPR and should have an emergency plan in the event of a serious injury.

A trained coach will know that she should:

- Structure a practice session to include conditioning exercises and warm-up and cool-down periods to lessen the incidence of related injuries.
- Give ample rest periods and water breaks to prevent overheating.
- Conduct a preseason conditioning program so athletes are fit and strong enough to play the sport.
- Not push kids to the point where they injure themselves.
- Discourage tactics like face blocking in football and sliding into base in baseball or softball.
- Ensure that the team has proper equipment and facilities.

- Enforce the wearing of protective equipment.
- Recognize early signs of pain and dysfunction in young athletes.
- Perform first aid or CPR if an accident occurs.
- Discourage unsafe practices such as crash diets and steroids.
- Provide appropriate motivation.

Isn't it obvious how important it is to have a trained coach in charge of your child? However, only about 20 percent of our volunteer coaches have any formal training. That percentage must rise if we hope to reduce the incidence of injuries in children's sports.

The pre-sports physical exam is another important aspect of injury prevention. The physician should look for conditions that might predispose your child to injury. For example, loose-jointed children may be susceptible to injuries in contact sports and should probably be directed toward sports such as track and field or rowing. At the opposite extreme, youngsters with very tight ligaments also have an increased risk of injury, particularly to the pelvis, hips, and spine. Unfortunately, many community-based sports programs don't even require an examination prior to participation. I am confident that as sports medicine takes a more prominent place in our culture, this situation will change. In the meantime, you must make sure that your child gets a comprehensive physical before he starts a sports program.

Because of children's vulnerability to growth plate injuries, I'm strongly in favor of making rule changes in organized sports to decrease the rates of injury. Some good changes that have been made are the Little League pitching limit of six innings a week and the prohibition of sliding; Pop Warner football did well to eliminate cross-body blocking or spearing. I've noticed a significant drop in certain trauma injuries due to these changes.

Another option that needs to be explored more fully in the collision sports is matching kids by size rather than just by age.

Just consider that boys in junior high range in weight from seventy-five to over two hundred pounds and can be anywhere from four and a half feet tall to a towering six feet! Physical mismatches occur when insufficient time and effort goes into organizing athletic programs and kids are divided by age alone. Disparities in size and weight can cause injury rates to soar. I've talked to some kids who are smaller than their peers who have been frightened to enter football programs because of size and weight differences. However, when placed in a program with similarly proportioned children, these kids have played football safely and successfully. Football is a great sport, and it shouldn't be restricted to the giants among us.

Proper conditioning is certainly an effective way to prevent unnecessary injuries. You should make sure your child is fit and strong enough for the sport she's going to play by asking the team coach for a preseason conditioning program. Unfit kids who are exhausted during a game are far more likely to trip and sprain an ankle or even sustain a growth plate fracture than those who are fit. Overweight children are predisposed to injuries, mainly because their growing bones are unable to withstand the stress of their extra weight.

A program to build strength and flexibility can enhance children's resistance to injury. Weight training to build strength has traditionally been viewed with skepticism by athletes in non-power sports because of concerns that it causes one to be "muscle bound." Not true! If it's done right, weight training actually improves flexibility (see Chapter 8). Concerns about whether weightlifting will cause growth plate fractures have also been put to rest. Under proper supervision, using the low-weight, high-repetition technique, they run no significant risk of injury.

Sports injuries are less likely to occur if your child is using proper equipment and facilities.* These include:

—————

*Minimum standards for athletic equipment are provided by the National Op-

- Playing fields free of potholes, glass, or other debris
- Padded posts
- Proper footwear
- Well-fitted protective padding and head gear
- Equipment sized for child athletes, including hockey sticks, baseball bats, tennis rackets, and skis
- Enforced wearing of safety equipment such as mouthguards, cups, and flotation jackets

A preseason meeting between parents and program organizers will allow you to voice your concerns about equipment and facilities. Make your feelings known!

One of the best ways to prevent injuries is for coaches and parents to encourage a relaxed attitude toward sports. Children shouldn't be obsessed with being the biggest, the fastest, and the best. In some sports — football, hockey, and baseball, for example — players are often encouraged to play and train too intensely. They are at greater risk of injury, including irreversible injury to a growth plate. The young runner or swimmer may sustain an overuse injury if he's pushed to train too hard; the football lineman, because of the "win at all cost" attitude drummed into his head by an irresponsible coach, may be playing too hard. Kids must be able to enjoy sports without being pressured too hard to win.

Catastrophic Injury: A Parent's Worst Fear

At the back of every parent's mind lurks the fear that a youngster involved in a contact sport will sustain a catastrophic injury.

---

erating Committee on Standards for Athletic Equipment and the American National Standards Institute (see the Appendix, under "Health, Fitness, and Safety," for addresses and phone numbers).

For those of us in sports medicine with an athletic background in football, hockey, or rugby, this is an especially gut-wrenching issue. Most of us come down on the side of participation, but only if all the appropriate precautions are taken. Of course, if you decide that you don't want your child to run the one in a million chance of sustaining a fatal or disabling injury, then no responsible physician would try to change your mind. Any sports-related fatality is a tragedy, and we must work to reduce the number of such accidents. What parents can do on their own is to make sure that a child who is going to participate in a collision sport gets a comprehensive physical exam and that he undertakes a conditioning program to strengthen vulnerable areas, especially the neck.

It's worth noting that the catastrophic injury rate in football is declining rapidly. High school football during the 1987 season experienced the lowest number of deaths since 1931. According to Frederick O. Mueller, director of the National Center for Catastrophic Injury Research, the 1960s was the worst decade for high school football fatalities. In 1968 there were thirty-six football deaths. From 1975 to 1988, however, profound changes in the sport reduced the number of catastrophic injuries. Mueller cites the following reasons for this welcome reduction:

1. Data collection allowed sports care professionals — physicians, coaches, athletic trainers, and others — to observe trends, investigate areas of concern, and carry out preventive measures. Reliable data are necessary for continued progress in preventing football injuries.

2. In 1968 the National Operating Committee on Standards in Athletic Equipment (NOCSAE) was founded to establish safety standards for athletic equipment. The initial effort was in head protection for football players. A safety standard for football helmets was set in 1973, and the first NOCSAE Standard helmets were tested the following year. The NOCSAE Standard was accepted by the National College Athletic Association (NCAA) in the 1978 football season and by the National Federation of

State High School Associations (NFSHA) in the 1980 season. All college and high school football players now must wear a NOC-SAE-certified football helmet.

3. Rule changes regarding safety have played a major role in reducing fatalities and disability injuries. The most significant change was the 1976 rule prohibiting initial contact with a player's helmet or face mask when tackling or blocking. The American Football Coaches Association (AFCA) Ethics Committee went on record opposing this now-illegal type of blocking and tackling, and their report is part of the football rules book.

4. Both high schools and colleges are making special efforts to coach their players in correct methods of tackling and blocking. This, along with safety education of coaches, has helped decrease head and neck injuries. Research in the laboratory and on the playing field has shown that the safest way to tackle and block is with the head held up rather than as the initial point of contact.

5. Coaches are emphasizing good physical conditioning, which helps reduce injuries. Coaches are also purchasing improved equipment and are placing more emphasis on proper fit of equipment, especially the helmet. Helmet manufacturers have stressed proper fit as a factor in reducing injuries.

6. Improved medical care of players has reduced injuries. Having a physician or athletic trainer on the field during both practice and play has helped prevent many injuries. Physicians are able to spot possible injuries and, by providing immediate care, often can prevent a minor injury from developing into something more serious. Some college programs have a physician *and* an athletic trainer at all games and practices. Many smaller programs have an athletic trainer on duty and a physician on call. Most states are setting the goal of having a qualified athletic trainer at each high school, though much more needs to be done in this direction.

Medical Coverage on the Playing Field

Almost nothing rivals the heart-stopping panic felt by a parent seeing her child go down on the field with a scream. In the vast majority of cases the child is immediately up and running and no worse for wear. But in many instances informed first aid and injury management are essential. First aid is a must not only in cases of spinal injury or heat stroke, but also in the less dramatic cases of twisted knees, cuts, and mild concussions. Mistakenly allowing an injured child to continue playing can have disastrous short- and long-term consequences. The slightly sprained ankle sustained by a young lacrosse player who plays on may soon require surgery; a concussion on the football field that goes unrecognized can be fatal if the player receives another blow to the head.

Unfortunately, most children's sports programs are woefully unprepared to provide even basic first aid, let alone cope with a medical emergency. This stems partly from society's attitude that sports injuries are unavoidable and don't require special attention. Many children who sustain injuries aren't managed properly. I can't tell you how many fractured ankles I've had to operate on because the fracture was initially dismissed as a sprain. More tragically, many children die or are severely disabled every year from neck injuries because no one on the spot knows what to do. "Do we take him to the hospital?" "We shouldn't move him, though, should we?" These are the panic-stricken questions asked by helpless onlookers. Standards of medical treatment in high school sports, which are subject to state law, are uneven at best. Not all states, for example, require that school sports coaches have first aid training.* And in community sports programs

*Those states that do not require coaches to have first aid training are Hawaii,

medical coverage is downright inadequate. There is no requirement that coaches in community sports programs have *any* first
aid training. With more and more children participating in community programs, this is a completely unacceptable state of affairs.

What level of medical coverage is needed in the sports program in which your youngster is enrolled? Although a fully
qualified sports medicine physician backed up by a team of EMTs
would cover all eventualities, most community health-care systems would resist providing this kind of coverage for all children's sports programs. In many cases they'd be right. For instance, I don't think that every Little League or Pop Warner
game needs its own five-person medical team sitting on the sidelines waiting for your nine-year-old to trip and twist her knee.
Let's be frank: at this level such extensive medical coverage would
be overkill. On the other hand, a certified athletic trainer or physician should be present at all high school football games, and
EMTs should be present or on call. Similarly, a gymnastics class
must always have someone available who knows what to do in an
emergency.

Ideally, every community sports program should have a medical coverage committee comprising five or six parents. If possible, two of them should have knowledge in sports medicine
and emergency medical care, say a doctor and a nurse or EMT.
This committee should determine what level of medical care is
required at games and organize that coverage. For an adolescent
football program, they would probably recommend that the coach
be trained in first aid and CPR to handle accidents in training,
that an athletic trainer or physician be present at games and, if
possible, an ambulance and EMT be on the premises during
competition. For Little League baseball or Pop Warner football,

---

Indiana, Maine, Massachusetts, Michigan, Nebraska, New Hampshire, North
Dakota, Ohio, Oregon, Pennsylvania, Rhode Island, and Vermont.

a coach with first aid training and an emergency plan is satisfactory.

However, it's unrealistic to expect each community program to have its own medical committee, though this is certainly a goal we must strive for. An acceptable alternative is for the community program's organizers to seek advice from their local chapter of the American College of Sports Medicine (ACSM).* The local chapter is also able to provide information to schools about medical coverage. Many state medical societies have sports medicine committees that are happy to dispense advice on this subject. Your primary care physician will know how to contact your state medical society. If the organizers of your youngster's sports program drag their feet on this matter, find out yourself what level of medical coverage is necessary. If it isn't being provided, get together with other parents and demand it.

In most cases someone in your child's sports environment should be qualified to provide triage. This is the decision-making process that occurs right after an accident to determine what action should be taken. For example, if your youngster scalds herself in the kitchen, you have to decide whether to take her to the hospital yourself or call the ambulance. That's triage. In a high school lacrosse game, a player leaves the field with a wrist injury, and the person providing triage must decide whether the wrist is fractured or sprained and whether the injured athlete should go to the hospital or be treated using the RICE technique (Rest, Ice, Compression, and Elevation).

Your local ACSM chapter or the state medical society's sports medicine committee should be able to provide you with the names of people willing and qualified to provide triage at children's sports events. The same person should be knowledgeable in first aid and CPR. An EMT is the best person for this job. The charge

*To find out how to contact your local ACSM chapter, write or call national headquarters: P.O. Box 1440, Indianapolis, Ind. 46206–1440. Phone (317) 637-9200.

is usually about fifty dollars, but when divided among the parents of thirty soccer players, let's say, that cost is worth the protection, in my view.

Ideally, the triage person should be available throughout the sports season. She need not necessarily be a physician. However, she should establish that she is in charge, should be prepared to handle acute injuries like a sprained wrist or broken ankle, and should be able to act quickly in a life-threatening emergency. The triage person also should determine if and when an injured athlete may return to play. She should have a working knowledge of common athletic injuries, of the signs that the child should be removed from play, and of the indications for hospitalization and observation. If possible, a quiet, well-lit room close to the playing and practice fields should be available for examination, first aid, and minor treatment like stitching a cut or bandaging an ankle.

It's important to have a plan for contacting an emergency medical facility if necessary. You'll need to have a telephone close to the sidelines or in a lockbox nearby, with keys for the triage person and two other adults in positions of responsibility. If such a setup is not possible, any parent with a portable cellular phone should inform the triage person of this well in advance of the game. If an ambulance or other emergency vehicle isn't available or necessary for the injury in question, then a parent with a station wagon should be available to act as the backup.

When an injury occurs, the triage person should go onto the field and determine whether the player should walk or be carried upright or on a stretcher to the examining area; be treated on the spot or wait until emergency care arrives; be allowed to continue playing immediately or after a short rest. The triage person should inform the coach as soon as the diagnosis and decision are made. *Under no circumstances should parents who want their child to continue playing contradict the triage person's decision.*

As most sports medicine experts will tell you, in the absence of a triage person, the individual best qualified to make decisions is the team coach. However, only a small minority of our millions of volunteer coaches have any first aid or CPR training. Mandatory coaching certification, as I've said, will improve this situation. Having coaches who can recognize serious but subtle injuries, as well as deal effectively with medical emergencies will help safeguard the health of our children during competition, as well as at practice, where at least half of all injuries occur. If the coach is not certified, at the very least he should have an emergency plan, and parents should ask to see it.

However, coaches should not have to shoulder the entire burden of learning first aid, CPR, and triage. Parents of sports-active children should take courses in first aid and CPR and, if need be, assume responsibility for providing such care in their child's sports program. Don't forget, first aid and CPR aren't important just in children's sports; they can also be vital in your own sports activities. For example, eye injuries are common in racket sports, and heat exhaustion occurs frequently in dance and aerobic classes. Would you know what to do if your spouse were hit square in the eye with a tennis ball? What would you do during an aerobics class if a friend became hot and dry, turned beet-red, and started acting irrationally? If you don't know the answers to these very common scenarios, then you need to learn much more about first aid. I strongly urge you to call your local American Red Cross office as soon as possible to ask about first aid courses.* I also suggest your youngsters take a first aid course as soon as they're old enough. Quite simply, first aid is a must for everybody!

*The American Red Cross is initiating courses in first aid for sports in a few states. This is a welcome step. Ask your local Red Cross office whether such a course is available in your area.

Handling Sports Injuries

When a child is injured in sports, the first decision is whether he requires medical attention and, if so, what kind. A sports accident can be a frightening experience, especially for a younger child, and he may burst into tears, causing you to think he is seriously injured when in fact he's just scared. It's important to have the child sit down for a few minutes. Often the tears will stop, and he will clamor to return to the fray.

However, if he has a real injury, it's important to act promptly and efficiently. In the following circumstances an injured child must be immediately taken to the closest hospital emergency room:

- Obvious deformity of any bone
- Localized tenderness or pain, especially in a joint
- Any alteration in consciousness
- Drowsiness
- Disorientation
- Persistent vomiting
- Pupils of unequal size
- Leakage of clear fluid from nose or ears
- Eye injury involving altered vision
- Seizure

Emergency First Aid

All parents should be familiar with the fundamentals of emergency first aid. Thankfully, most sports-related children's injuries are relatively minor. But certainly adults must be prepared for accidents.

Loss of consciousness, usually due to a head injury, is not uncommon in sports or free play. The cause might be a "bean ball," two kids knocking heads in soccer, or hitting the head against a goal post. The situation should be judged an emergency if the child doesn't respond when she is called by name in a loud voice, tapped on the chest and shaken gently, or is unresponsive or unaware of the surroundings. The face, gums, and inner eyelids may be flushed, white, or blue, depending on the cause of unconsciousness.

The child in this condition shouldn't be moved, and no further attempt should be made to rouse her. Someone should immediately call a medical facility for help. In the meantime, her clothing should be loosened, especially around the neck and waist. The child's legs should be raised, and her head turned to one side to encourage drainage of saliva and prevent choking. *If a serious head or neck injury is suspected, do not move the child at all.* Even if she regains consciousness, keep her lying down until medical attention arrives. Check for any signs of bleeding. If bleeding seems severe, apply strong, sustained pressure with a compress, clean cloth, or bare hand.

Carefully monitor the child's pulse. This is done most easily at the carotid artery, the major blood vessel in the neck. To find the carotid artery, place two or three fingers on the child's Adam's apple and slide your fingers sideways into the gap between the Adam's apple and the neck muscles. If the pulse stops, someone who is trained in CPR should begin this procedure immediately. If you can feel a pulse but the child is *not* breathing, artificial respiration should be started right away. Check the child's mouth and carefully remove any obstruction such as a mouthguard or bubble gum. Breathing may have stopped because she has inhaled water, mud, or some other substance. If her lips are blue, she is not getting oxygen. Obstruction of the airway is the most common cause of death in an unconscious child.

If the child's chest is rising and falling, even with difficulty, and you can feel her breath on your face, then she is breathing despite partial blockage of the airway. In such cases, it's best to transport the child as quickly as possible to a hospital emergency room. But if her lips are blue and she doesn't respond to gentle shaking and calling, immediately try to open the airway.

That may be all that's needed to restore breathing. To prevent the tongue from blocking the airway, lay the child on her back and tilt the head up slightly. If the child doesn't begin coughing or struggling to breathe within a few seconds after opening the airway, someone trained in artificial respiration must attempt to breathe for her until medical help arrives. Continue to check for a pulse. If the child begins coughing or breathing independently before help arrives, keep her calm by speaking in a slow, reassuring way. If the child doesn't begin breathing independently, the pulse may also stop, and CPR should begin and be continued while transporting the child.

Common Sports Injuries

Sprains and strains. A sprain is a partial or complete tear in a ligament, one of the ropelike tissues that connect the bones and give strength and stability to our joints. A common ligament sprain is a sprained ankle. A strain is an overstretched muscle. Quadricep and hamstring strains are two of the most common.

Sprains and strains can be classified as: first degree, or mild; second degree, or moderate; and third degree, or serious. If your foot slips on the stairs and you feel a sharp twinge as the ligaments stretch, but not to the point of tearing, you may have a first-degree ankle sprain. If your arms feel sore the day after you've moved to a new house, you may have suffered a first-degree muscle strain of the biceps. Children who sustain first-degree sprains or strains usually won't want or need to stop playing. If they do stop, they can return to play after fifteen minutes if the pain subsides and they have full range of motion in the affected area. To determine whether a child may return to action, see if she can do a push-up (in the case of an arm sprain or strain) or jump up and down (in the case of a leg sprain or strain). If swelling develops after the game, it can be treated with RICE (see the box on pages 94–95).

Second-degree sprains and strains range from a small tear to almost complete rupture of ligaments or muscles. Swelling, pain, and stiffness usually occur immediately. RICE, splinting, and examination by a qualified physician at a nearby hospital are essential.

Third-degree sprains and strains are complete tears of a ligament or muscle. Pain is felt immediately but may subside because the pain fibers aren't activated when ligaments and muscles are completely torn. Swelling may be negligible. Ironically, the most severe sprains and strains may produce the least pain and may thus be disregarded by the child and by an inexperienced or untrained coach. If a severe sprain or strain is suspected — loss of function is the giveaway sign — the injured area should be stabilized and the child removed from the playing field and taken to the closest hospital for X rays. Proper diagnosis and rehabilitation are essential.

Bruises. A bruise, or contusion, as it's known in medical terminology, is caused by impact to a muscle that causes bleeding under the skin. A bruise may be so slight as to go unnoticed until hours or days later, when you think, "How did I get that?" Or it may be so severe as to cause gross swelling, loss of function, and sharp or aching pain. A hard blow to the thigh, for example, an injury often sustained by football players and sometimes referred to as a "charley horse," can cause severe swelling. I've seen a thigh bruise permanently limit a soccer player's mobility, and a forearm bruise actually threaten the blood supply to a hockey player's hand because the swelling was so extensive.

All bruises are helped by RICE. Although heating pads or warm

RICE: The First Step in Injury Management

●

The first few minutes of care are crucial in reducing both the severity of the injury and the period of disability. For muscle-tendon injuries, a series of four traditional steps is particularly effective. The acronym RICE stands for Rest, Ice, Compression, and Elevation. Each step is essential.

Rest. In sports injuries rest is always relative. Any patient with a sports injury should have an exercise program aimed at restoring or maintaining function, and thus will not be strictly at rest. In this context rest means that the injury should not be abused. For example, a soccer player with a severe leg bruise must stop running, but I would urge him to swim an hour a day, six days a week, if this doesn't cause pain or recurrent swelling in the injured leg. This athlete, although not playing soccer, certainly is not "resting."

Ice. In the past, ice application was recommended for only twenty-four to forty-eight hours following the injury. Evidence now suggests that intermittent icing may be beneficial for up to seven days, particularly for severe bruises. The first seventy-two hours are especially critical, and icing should be done as much as is practically possible during this period, according to these guidelines.

Ice should be applied immediately after injury and is most effective when done intermittently; I prefer an ice massage technique. I instruct my patients to freeze water in several plastic foam coffee cups and then to tear off the upper edge of the cup. This leaves the base as an insulated grip, and enables them to massage the injured area in a circular pattern for ten to fifteen minutes at intervals of thirty to forty-five minutes.

Compression. All too often neglected during the early stages of injury management, compression should be gentle, so as not to cause pain. The most convenient method is to use elastic bandage. Children should be warned not to wrap the bandage too tightly, causing a tourniquet effect. Compression and cooling can be combined by using elastic bandages that have been

RICE: The First Step in Injury Management

●

stored in ice water, but the bandage should be removed at intervals for ice massage.

Elevation. The last component of RICE, elevation is often neglected or improperly performed. True hypodynamic elevation means raising the injured limb above heart level. Instead I often see athletes on the sidelines with an injured ankle or knee thrust out horizontally. Clearly, this isn't hypodynamic elevation, and it is a serious therapeutic error. The child should be instructed to sit in such a way that the blood flows downward, unimpeded, from the injured arm or leg to the heart.

These general measures should be used for the first twenty-four to forty-eight hours after an injury. Specific exercises or heat may be helpful later to restore strength and function after a sports injury, but it can be harmful to use them prematurely, particularly for young athletes.

whirlpools may improve range of motion and comfort, if they are used too soon after the injury these techniques can cause further bleeding and worsen the bruising. Severe bruising must be treated by a physician. When I see a severe bruise, I feel it's best to err on the side of caution and apply ice intermittently for five to seven days.

Fractures. Occasionally you hear someone ask, "Is it a break or a fracture?" They are one and the same. Any blow great enough to cause severe bruising in a child may also cause the underlying bone to fracture, even if the bone does not show deformity. The guideline used to be that if an athlete could walk on an injured leg or use an injured arm, there was no break. However, this isn't an accurate guideline. Sometimes the fractured limb can be used. The problem is, if a fracture is mistaken for, and treated as, a sprain, serious problems usually result. A better way to tell whether a child has sustained a fracture if there is no obvious deformity is to compare the range of motion with that of the opposite limb and check for swelling at the joint. But if there is any doubt, seek medical assessment.

If a fracture is suspected, the limb should be splinted before the athlete is moved. The splint should include the joint above and below the injury. Highly sophisticated splints have been developed to fit knees, ankles, or wrists, but as anyone who has taken a first aid course knows, a perfectly satisfactory splint can be made from heavy cardboard, a padded magazine, or a cane. When making a makeshift splint, be sure it is well padded and the bandages aren't too tight. Check the circulation in the child's fingers and toes by seeing if they are pink and warm. The splint should make the injured limb more comfortable, and if it isn't doing this, it should be removed. Any open wound should be covered with a sterile dressing from the medical kit. After these measures are taken, the child should be transported to the hospital.

Cuts. Blood can be a frightening sight for both athletes and parents. But if handled properly, cuts are rarely serious. Small cuts and scrapes can be patched up by someone with rudimentary first aid training, and the athlete returned to action. Obviously, the care of large or open wounds is a different story. These require serious attention. Bleeding should be controlled by gently applying gauze from the medical kit. After the bleeding slows, the wound should be sterilized to avoid contamination. If a medical person is not on hand to sew stitches, the child should be taken to the nearest hospital emergency room.

Concussion. A blow to the head can cause damage to the brain tissue, known as concussion. Managing concussion properly is often difficult because there may be no visible signs. In the hurly-burly of competition, a concussion is often mismanaged, occasionally with tragic consequences. If a concussed child is allowed to continue playing and receives another blow to the head, he may go into a coma or even die. This is known as "second impact syndrome." It's very important to go out of our way to detect concussions in sports.

Concussions fall into three main categories. A first-degree, or mild, concussion makes the athlete feel confused and dazed and experience slight amnesia. To detect mild concussion, ask the child what the score is, what day it is, or how she got to the field that day. Any hesitation in answering any of these questions probably means the child is mildly concussed. Second-degree, or moderate, concussion may cause unconsciousness for a few seconds or several minutes. Third-degree, or severe, concussion means any lapse of consciousness for more than five minutes.

Although it is extremely rare, spinal injury should always be assumed in the case of second- or third-degree concussion. Until spinal injury is ruled out, the game must stop and the child must not be moved. His breathing and pulse should be checked (see "Emergency First Aid") while someone calls a hospital and an ambulance. If pulse and breathing are normal, wait for the child to regain consciousness. If, on regaining consciousness, the child complains of neck or back pain or of numbness in the arms or legs, *don't move him!* If all is normal, wait until the player is ready to move and assist him to a kneeling position. When he is able to stand, help him to his feet and assist him to the sideline, carefully watching his progress. If the athlete can't walk, call for a stretcher or litter. If necessary, halt the game until an ambulance arrives.

An athlete who sustains a concussion, however mild, must not return to play until cleared by a physician.

Heat injuries. Children have inefficient thermoregulatory systems, which means they are unable to cope with heat as well as adults and are therefore susceptible to the two types of heat-related disorders: heat exhaustion and the much more serious heat stroke. These two conditions are often confused.

Heat exhaustion is caused by dehydration and salt loss. Children with heat exhaustion become cool and damp while running a normal temperature, and often feel dizzy and tired. They should be given plenty of fluids and should rest in a cool, shady place with their clothing loosened.

Heat stroke is caused by a disruption of the body's thermoregulatory mechanism. The athlete becomes hot and dry, turns beet-red, and runs a high fever. He or she may also act irrationally, often aggressively. Heat stroke must be treated by rapidly cooling the athlete with ice water, towels soaked in ice cold water, and fanning. Any child who suffers heat stroke should be taken to the hospital immediately for observation.

Head-to-Toe First Aid Scenarios

Head

As he tackles an opponent, a high school football player's head snaps forward, causing him to lose consciousness.

During a soccer game, an eleven-year-old collides head first with another youngster and goes down holding his head.

A fourteen-year-old diver attempts a backward somersault and cuts her head on the diving board.

Head and neck injuries must be taken very seriously. If a child complains of any neck or back pain, or more significantly, numbness or weakness in the arms or legs, she must not be moved except by a qualified medical person. Any signs of concussion mean the child must not return to play without a physician's ok. Some common-sense criteria for removing a child with a head or neck injury from play are the following: "seeing stars," dizziness, ringing in the ears, nausea, vomiting, severe headache, amnesia, confusion, unequal pupils, and weakness or numbness anywhere in the body.

Head wounds often bleed profusely, but they usually stop

bleeding soon. Gauze from the medical kit should be pressed gently against the cut. If the child will not be receiving medical attention at a hospital right away, then ice should also be applied to the area.

Eye

A junior high soccer goalkeeper dives at the feet of an oncoming player and receives a kick just below the eye.

Eye injuries are common and must be treated with the greatest respect. Always check first for signs of concussion. A black eye, or "shiner," has become a badge of courage in our society, and young boys love showing one off. Perhaps as a result, they often are not treated seriously enough. Long-term damage can be caused by an injury that people dismiss as "just a black eye." One such injury is *hyphemia,* in which blood collects in the anterior chamber of the eye, causing pain and changes in vision. A child who suffers an eye injury that causes pain, blurred vision, or sensitivity to light should have the injured eye closed and covered with a soft dressing held in place with a bandage. The child must be immediately removed from the playing field and taken to a qualified physician or ophthalmologist.

Nose

A Little League first baseman gets hit in the nose by a ball thrown by the second basewoman.

Check first to see whether there is any concussion. To stop a bloody nose, have the youngster sit up, and gently squeeze the nostrils. Do not tilt the head back. If the nose doesn't stop bleeding in fifteen minutes, the athlete should be driven to the closest hospital emergency room.

Teeth

A hockey goalkeeper has half of a front tooth knocked out by a flying puck.

If a tooth is broken or knocked out, it should be put into a container with milk, saliva, or salt water but *not washed* — this kills the tooth, which otherwise may be reaffixed. The youngster should be taken to an emergency room, along with the tooth, and assessed by a physician, dentist, or oral physician.

Ear

A junior high wrestler develops a "cauliflower ear."

Preparing to hit a home run, an eleven-year-old baseball player is hit on the ear by a wild pitch.

Trauma injuries of the ear should be treated with intermittent icing and compression. A cauliflower ear, which involves swelling between the cartilaginous part of the ear and the skin, caused by frequent rubbing, should be examined by a physician. If there is any hearing loss or ringing in the ears, the child should be referred to an ear specialist.

Chest

During a high school championship hockey game, a player receives a blow to the chest.

Chest injuries can be very dangerous. Any child who complains of pain or shortness of breath must be taken to the nearest hospital emergency room. Tragically, chest injuries are sometimes mismanaged, and several deaths a year occur because fluid collects around the heart or a lung is punctured by a broken rib.

Abdomen

A young football quarterback gets "speared" in the stomach by an oncoming lineman.

Any child who receives a blow to the abdomen should be removed from play for at least fifteen minutes. If the player is just winded, he can then return to action. However, if there is any tenderness or, more significantly, symptoms such as dizziness, paleness, vomiting, a distended stomach, a rapid pulse, clamminess, or sweating, the youngster must be taken immediately to the closest hospital emergency room.

Arms and Legs

Springing to catch a fly ball, a Little League outfielder trips and sprains an ankle.

A seventeen-year-old football player is tackled and feels a sharp crack in his thighbone.

Losing her balance on the beam, a twelve-year-old gymnast falls awkwardly and feels her shoulder "pop out."

The first step when managing an arm or leg injury is to determine its severity. If there are clear signs that a bone is broken, such as an obvious deformity, the limb should be gently splinted and the child taken to the hospital. If there are no signs of obvious deformity, the youngster should rest for fifteen minutes, using the RICE technique on the affected area. After fifteen minutes the child should be tested for pain and range of motion. To test the arms, ask the child to do a wall push-up; for the legs, ask the child to jump up and down. If the range of motion is restricted or there is pain, then the child must be examined by a physician.

To Sum Up

Injuries that are not treated may keep children from participating in sports in the short term and, if serious, may hinder their future participation and all-around health. A simple technique such as RICE for a sprained ankle can make the difference between quick recovery and being out for two weeks or a month. Parents must take their children's complaints of pain seriously and make sure they get proper medical attention.

Let's not forget about prevention. We've seen several clear ways to minimize the potential for injuries in children's sports. In fact, this is the real issue — not whether injuries will occur in children's sports, but whether *unnecessary* injuries happen. At present, far too many trauma injuries are preventable. So let's ditch the old saw that children's sports injuries are "just part of the game" and work to prevent their occurrence.

The nonprofit National Youth Sports Foundation for the Prevention of Athletic Injuries (NYSFPAI), of which I am a director, has formulated a comprehensive list of safety measures for children's sports:

- Athletes and parents should know the inherent dangers of the sports the children are playing.
- Athletes should have a pre-sports physical by a sports medicine specialist.
- Athletes should have an off-season and preseason conditioning program. The plan should be designed by a person with training in exercise physiology and directed by the coach.
- Athletes should perform warm-up and cool-down exercises led by their coach.
- Athletes can choose not to play if they are injured and feel there is a risk of further injury to themselves.
- Athletes should be coached by adults with at least a minimum level of competence in the sport and a knowledge of injury

prevention, conditioning, exercise physiology, and psychology.

- Athletes should be coached by someone with first aid and CPR training and an emergency plan in case of serious injury.
- Athletes should play in a safe facility.
- Athletes should have approved safety equipment that fits properly.

5

•••••

Overuse Injuries:
The New Problem

Acute sports injuries such as the ones described in the previous chapter are well known to the medical profession. Now we're learning about a whole new genre of children's sports injuries — overuse injuries.

It's been said that no horse ever ran itself to death until it had a rider on its back. Similarly, no child ever did anything repetitive enough in a sandlot game to cause an overuse injury. There's no question that overuse injuries are a direct outgrowth of the organization of children's sports. Shin splints, swimmer's shoulder, and gymnast's back are but three common overuse injuries that used to be unheard of in children. Now they're buzzwords in the youth sports lexicon, not to mention in the corridors of sports clinics around the country. Overuse injuries such as stress fractures, tendinitis, bursitis, and joint disorders, once thought to be the preserve of adult athletes, are now commonplace in children's athletic programs. Consider the fact that overuse knee injuries like *patellar pain syndrome* were rarely seen in children until a quarter century ago, when vigorous sports programs for children began in earnest. It's now the number-one diagnosis in my clinic! Stress fractures in young athletes have reached similar epidemic proportions.

Overuse injuries result from repetitive microtrauma to tissues, caused by activities such as overhead hurling in baseball, tennis, volleyball, and javelin; the pounding of feet against the ground in running and dancing; and repeated flexion and extension of the back in gymnastics, diving, and dancing. Unlike acute injuries, which occur in both organized sports and free play, overuse injuries have the dubious honor of being exclusive to organized sports. In that respect, they are true sports injuries.

In the free play that once dominated American children's leisure time, kids who were hurt went home and usually didn't return to play until they felt better. But children in organized sports often overtrain and may even play when hurt. Part of the problem is that amateur coaches are unaware of the special vulnerability of children to overuse injuries and unknowingly push them too hard. And because of the pressures of organized programs, kids will often conceal a sore elbow or an aching knee because they don't want to look like sissies. A child with swimmer's shoulder told me last week that he had suppressed the pain because he didn't want to look like a "wimp" in front of the coach and his teammates. Unfortunately, the injury, untreated, had progressed to the stage where I was forced to refer him for surgery.

Not only are our children asked to perform the rigorous, repetitive sports tasks of modern adult sports, but they are pressured to perform them at the expense of all other activities. Indeed, the rise of young sports specialists has been closely tied to the growing number of overuse injuries. Rather than play whatever sport is in season, as many of us did as kids, these athletes choose their sport at an early age and train exclusively in that one or perhaps two sports year-round. Such training subjects the young athlete to the continual microtrauma that causes overuse injury.

Two aspects of this phenomenon are especially troubling to me. First, overuse injuries are prevalent in the lifetime sports such as jogging, cycling, swimming, and aerobic dance, which rely on repetitive movements of large muscle groups. These sports are essential for lifelong health fitness, but a severe overuse injury can render future participation impossible because of the potential for reinjury. I recently had to operate on a young soccer player to repair the inside of her kneecap which was completely worn away. She will always be predisposed to knee pain when running. In some cases the injury is never diagnosed, and the youngster simply drops out of all health fitness activities and goes on to lead a sedentary life. I have encountered several young adults who claimed that they didn't play sports or do any fitness activities because as kids they were "always getting injured." But after asking them a few questions, it turned out that they had suffered overuse injuries that had never been diagnosed, which led them to believe their bodies were "naturally weak."

Ironically, the lifetime sports have been thought of as safe compared to sports like hockey, football, soccer, and basketball because the chances of acute injury are slim. For example, the mother of a five-year-old beginning athlete said to me the other day, "My kid's going to be a swimmer because I don't want him to be a football player and be injured half the time." She was correct in thinking that her son wouldn't be exposed to the "brutishness" (her word, not mine) of football, but mistaken to assume he was being sheltered from all injuries. If this young fellow decides to take up swimming competitively, he'll have to watch out for overuse injuries of the knee and shoulder. Fortunately, most overuse injuries are preventable; if this mother takes the appropriate steps, the chances of her son sustaining an overuse injury will be minimized (see below, "Preventing Overuse Injuries").

Second, there is growing evidence that overuse injuries sustained in childhood may continue to cause problems in later life. I'm concerned that twenty or thirty years from now an unprecedented number of adults will have medical conditions — arthritis, for example — that we'll find were caused by overuse injuries in childhood.

When I diagnose an overuse injury in a child, I don't fault the sport. I fault our society for not introducing an effective system to prevent such injuries. Later in this chapter I'll discuss the measures needed to create such a system, including improving standards of coaching; making sure that all children get a presports physical; making sure our kids are fit; and simply listening to and respecting kids when they express the first signs of pain. But before we talk about prevention, it's important to learn the reasons why children are vulnerable to overuse injury.

The Growth Factor

Until quite recently, overuse injuries were seen only in adults, most often highly trained elite athletes and "weekend warriors" — sedentary adults who do no athletic activity during the week and then play three sets of tennis on Sunday. Because of this pattern, physicians thought that overuse injuries like tennis elbow resulted from too much stress on aging bones, muscles, tendons, and ligaments in a short period of time. However, with the rise of rigorous, repetitive sports training regimens for children, we've discovered that children are even more likely than adults to sustain these overuse syndromes.

Ask me if your kids are predisposed to overuse injuries, and my answer is always a resounding "Yes!" Children are more susceptible than adults to overuse injury because growth is the fundamental feature of childhood. Growth makes kids vulnerable to overuse injuries for two reasons: the presence of growth cartilage and the growth process itself.

Growth Cartilage

This is a soft, thick layer of new bone cartilage waiting to harden into bone. It is found in three main sites in the growing child's body: the growth plates near the ends of the long bones; the cartilage lining the joint surfaces (articular cartilage); and the points at which the major tendons attach to the bones. Until your child stops growing, growth cartilage is present, and it is more easily damaged by repetitive microtrauma than thin, hard, fully formed adult bone cartilage. And because this cartilage is "bone waiting to happen," injuring it may have serious consequences in later life.

Repetitive microtrauma to the growth plates of the long bones, especially during running and dancing, can weaken the plate and cause the ball of the joint to slip. Displacement of the ball of the hip joint, a *slipped capital femoral epiphysis,* is the most common of these injuries. Overweight children are prime candidates for this condition. Surgery is almost always required to correct a slipped ball of the hip joint, which, if undetected, can cause arthritis in later life. Tiny fractures to the growth plate of the ball of the shoulder joint, best known as Little League shoulder, are common in baseball players. Usually rest will take care of this condition. A *vertebral growth-plate fracture,* a stress fracture to the vulnerable growth plates of the vertebrae caused by repetitive bending, is a common back injury sustained by child athletes. This condition is sometimes known as *Schuermann's disease* when it occurs at the top of the back and atypical Schuermann's disease in the lower back, as it is more frequently in kids. Gymnasts, oarsmen, and divers are especially vulnerable to this injury because of the characteristic bending motions of these activities. Vertebral growth-plate fractures are usually treated successfully with bracing, rest, and an exercise program to correct the "sway-back" that often contributes to this condition. If left untreated, vertebral growth-plate fractures can lead to spine deformities and persistent lifelong back pain, sometimes accompanied by arthritis.

The best-known overuse injury of the joint surface cartilage is Little League elbow, which can occur in any sport that requires a "whipping" overarm action, such as baseball, volleyball, tennis, and javelin. Unlike adults' pitcher's elbow or tennis elbow, which affects muscles and tendons, Little League elbow involves trauma to the growth cartilage itself, which of course is unformed bone. In adults the bones are stronger than soft tissues. But in children the muscles and tendons may be stronger than the growth cartilage, and the repetitive stress of overarm throwing can cause chips of it to break off and lodge in the elbow joint. These chips then enlarge and, like a monkey wrench thrown into machinery, eventually cause the elbow joint to lock in a given position. This causes excruciating pain and, unless the problem is recognized and managed in the early stages, long-term growth abnormalities in the bone, which may mean elbow pain and dysfunction for life. A child who complains of elbow pain must be treated immediately to avoid growth abnormalities. All throwing must cease for at least six to nine weeks to promote reattachment of the displaced growth cartilage. Surgery may be needed to ensure proper positioning of the bone during healing. In time the child may resume throwing, but only after he has been given a strengthening program for the whole arm and has been taught throwing technique that won't cause another episode.

Little League elbow is a household term because organized children's baseball has been with us since 1947. But distance running for children has emerged only in the last decade or so. It was once believed that children's hearts and lungs couldn't stand the physiological stress of endurance activities. However, it has been found that healthy children run no higher risk than adults of cardiovascular injury. Young ankles and knees are a different story. The knee is now the most common site of overuse injury in children. "Teenager's knee," known in medical terminology as *Osteochondritis dissecans,* a disorder unique to growing children, is a common overuse injury affecting the joint surface cartilage. Osteochondritis dissecans of the knee is caused by the repetitive bumping and grinding of the growth cartilage of the bottom end of the thighbone against the top of the shinbone. Because a child's joint cartilage is both thicker and softer than that of an adult, the force of repeated impact, as in running, is much more likely to cause a stress fracture. Eventually a divot forms on the joint surface, causing pain, swelling, and tenderness on the inside of the knee. If the problem isn't caught early enough, the damaged piece of cartilage falls off and floats around in the joint area, causing the knee joint to lock. This is different from the damage to the joint cartilage sustained in throwing, which is caused by the whipping motion shearing off chips of bone cartilage. Osteochondritis dissecans is caused by the impact of bones crunching together.

Treatment of this condition depends on whether the piece of cartilage has actually detached. If it hasn't, three to six months of rest may enable the divot to heal. In young athletes whose bones are still growing rapidly, the divot usually heals completely. But if after six months the child is still experiencing pain, and X rays show no sign of healing, then surgery may be required. In surgery I try to help the injury heal itself by drilling through the damaged piece into the healthy bone beneath and pinning the fragment in place to stimulate the rejoining process. When the piece has healed in place, the child must undertake a quadricep and hamstring strengthening program. After six months the patient should be ready to return to sports action.

If the piece of joint cartilage detaches completely from the end of the bone, the joint will usually lock. Almost always the knee swells and can't even be straightened. X rays clearly reveal the loose bone chips and crater, telling me that surgery is the only option. With an arthroscope (a pencil-sized telescopelike device that enables me to peer into the knee), I locate the loose pieces of cartilage and remove them. Then I drill a hole into the crater to stimulate blood flow, thus encouraging bone to grow and fill the gap. The rehabilitation program is identical to that for nondetached osteochondritis dissecans. Needless to say, losing a one-inch-square piece of your knee at age fourteen is best avoided and, with early detection, it can be.

Osteochondritis dissecans also occurs in the ankle from repetitive grinding of the growth cartilage at the bottom of the shinbone and the top of the anklebone. Treatment is the same as for this condition in the knee. Very occasionally, osteochondritis dissecans is seen in the hip.

The third site of especially vulnerable growth cartilage in children is the apophyses, the places where major tendons attach to bone. The best-known injury of this type occurs where the tendon from the kneecap attaches to the growth cartilage at the top of the shinbone. This condition goes by the name of *Osgood-Schlatter's disease,* although it isn't actually a disease. It occurs most often in kids between nine and fourteen years of age, and it appears as a lump at the top of the shinbone just below the knee. In about 20 percent of cases it is present in both knees. I see this condition most often when the sport season begins and kids train too hard after a period of relative inactivity. Although it usually begins as a low-grade ache felt when the child gets out of bed in the morning, an ache that probably won't discourage the enthusiastic young athlete from sports, after a fortnight it often develops into severe discomfort. At this point the child is unable to run at full speed and may limp when walking. The pain is especially acute when squatting, climbing stairs, or walking uphill. Traditionally, Osgood-Schlatter's disease was associated with active boys at the onset of the growth spurt, though with the increased opportunities for girls in sports we're now seeing many more girls with this condition. Despite its fearsome-sounding name, Osgood-Schlatter's disease is easily treated with a program of strength and flexibility exercises to alleviate the tightness of the tendons and allow the injury to heal.

Another common injury affecting the growth cartilage at the

major tendon insertions is "Seven's disease," *os calcis apophysitis,* felt as tenderness where the Achilles tendon meets the heel bone. As with Osgood-Schlatter's disease, the injury occurs when a child with tight calf muscles suddenly does a lot more running and jumping. Youngsters with this condition — often soccer and lacrosse players — usually respond well to a program of Achilles tendon stretching and ankle strengthening exercises.

The Growth Process

The major role of growth cartilage in predisposing kids to overuse injury is now well known in the medical community. What isn't as well recognized is that all overuse injuries are exacerbated by the growth process itself. For the past decade I've devoted an enormous amount of research time to unraveling the mysteries of growth and to discovering how and why it increases the risk of overuse injuries in children.

My research has identified the chief culprit: tightness in growing muscles and tendons. As bones grow, the muscles and tendons don't grow at the same rate but instead must stretch to keep up. During the adolescent growth spurt, the bones in your child's legs grow so quickly that a height increase of three quarters of an inch in a month is not uncommon. But because the muscles and tendons spanning these rapidly growing bones don't elongate as quickly, they get much tighter. The loss of flexibility increases the likelihood of overuse injuries, particularly in the powerful extensor mechanism of the knee — the combined structure of the quadriceps muscle, the kneecap, and the tendon attaching the kneecap to the shinbone, which allows the leg to perform all its dynamic movements.

A very common overuse injury occurs when the cartilage on the underside of the kneecap is irritated by the kneecap sliding over the bottom of the thighbone when the leg is repeatedly bent during physical activity. This injury is called *patellofemoral stress syndrome* and is characterized by pain in the kneecap. The pain worsens during knee-bending activities such as climbing stairs, sitting for extended periods, squatting, or kneeling. My treatment for this condition most often includes straight-leg strengthening exercises and a flexibility program for the hamstrings and quadriceps to alleviate the imbalances caused by the growth process. If the problem isn't taken care of, the surface cartilage under the kneecap may split or break up, a condiion called *chondromalacia patella.*

Bursitis of the hip, known as *trochanteric bursitis,* is an inflammation of the fluid-filled *bursa* on the outside of the hip joint. In adults, this condition may be caused by a blow, but in children it is usually caused by the growth-related tightness of the wide sheet of tendons that restrain the thigh muscles, the *iliotibial band.* This causes the bursa to become irritated and then inflamed. The condition is most often brought on by a sudden increase in intensity of a training program involving running and jumping. The usual symptom of trochanteric bursitis is a dull, painful ache that becomes acute when the area is even lightly probed. A clicking sensation may be felt over the bone, which is why this condition is sometimes known as snapping hip. Conservative treatment, including RICE, aspirin, and occasionally ultrasound, is the best approach to treating trochanteric bursitis. *Iliopsoas tendinitis* is the same condition on the inside of the hip near the groin. Special exercises to stretch the tendon of the iliopsoas muscle and strengthen adjacent muscles will usually eliminate the pain and "snapping."

Children are also vulnerable to overuse injuries of the lower back when the spine is growing faster than its muscles and tendons. The resulting tightness may even alter the child's posture, and such a change is likely to cause injuries. Lower-back pain is associated with swayback, or *lumbar lordosis,* as it's properly known. Tightly stretched back muscles, weak abdominal muscles, tight hip muscles, and weak hamstrings all combine to make the pelvis tilt forward and the shoulders tilt back. Some kids, boys especially, develop "roundback" in order to reposition the torso forward over the pelvis. Both swayback and roundback put immense pressure on the spine. A child who is developing this posture due to the growth process and is in sports training that involves repetitive stretching, bending, and rotating the spine, may show a characteristic pattern of injuries. All my research tells me that swayback and roundback are important contributors to several overuse back injuries involving disks and vertebrae. These include *spondylosis, spondylolisthesis, vertebral growth-plate fractures,* and *discogenic* pain (slipped disk). I have helped develop several back braces that I've used with a great deal of success to treat kids with back problems. However, in severe cases, surgery may be necessary.

Unlike acute injuries, such as sprained ankles, broken legs, and split lips, which are usually caused by a single event, overuse injuries usually result from a combination of risk factors (see the box on page 115). When I'm trying to determine the cause of a young athlete's overuse injury, I go through a check list of risk factors. My thought process goes something like this: Why would a fourteen-year-old figure skater sustain a stress fracture of her *left* foot? Was it her skates? her foot structure? her training? Why does a twelve-year-old ballet dancer develop a painful Achilles tendon in her *right* heel? Is it the floor surface? her knock-knees? a pushy instructor? Why does the fifteen-year-old cross-country runner, who's been running without problems since age ten, suddenly develop pain below *both* knees? Is it his shoes? his growth spurt? running on hills?

Unraveling these contributory factors is one of the greatest challenges facing the sports physician. It is essential that the injury be treated properly so that the tissue can heal and the child can resume athletic activity without recurrence of the condition. As you know, a broken arm caused by a fall from a tree is treated

Risk Factors for Overuse Injuries

●

Growth

Cultural deconditioning (lack of fitness)

Musculoskeletal weakness
Obesity

Training errors

Abrupt change in intensity, duration, or frequency of training
Imbalances of strength or flexibility in muscles and tendons

Anatomical malalignment of the legs

Differences in length
Abnormal position of the kneecap
Bowlegs, knock-knees, or flat feet

Improper footwear

Incorrect fit
Inadequate absorption of impact
Excessively stiff sole
Insufficient heel support

Hardness of playing or running surface

Associated disease, including old injuries

---

the same as a broken arm sustained in football. But it's much more difficult to assess, treat, and prevent the recurrence of an inflamed shoulder tendon in a twelve-year-old swimmer who wants to swim 8,000 yards a day to defend her state title in a month's time. Often the newest and most sophisticated diagnostic techniques — magnetic resonance imaging (MRI), CAT scans, EMGs, and the like — are necessary to make the proper diagnosis. For this reason, it is infinitely preferable to prevent overuse injuries than to treat them.

Preventing Overuse Injuries

I'm in surgery fifteen to twenty times a week, often to correct or alleviate overuse injuries. I have most child athletes back in action within a few months, thanks to modern diagnostic and surgical techniques, some of which I've pioneered. I often receive thank you letters from my young patients, but I know full well that they wish they had never met me, at least under those circumstances! Prevention is always better than cure, especially in the case of overuse injuries.

Overuse injuries are almost always preventable. They occur not as the result of an accident, as acute injuries do, but when kids do exactly what they're supposed to do — only they do it too much. Is your child's participation in organized sports compatible with avoiding overuse injuries? I say it is compatible, through a system with four components that are within the reach of all parents.

Qualified Adult Supervision

Probably the biggest problem facing our kids is that they're coached by unqualified adults who are simply unaware of children's vulnerability to overuse injury. Training error is one of the biggest culprits in causing overuse injuries. Little League elbow, the result of incorrect technique and simply throwing too much, is caused by improper training. The seventh grader who has never participated in organized sports and then makes the track team as a middle-distance runner is highly susceptible to overuse knee injuries in a poorly supervised training program. It's for this reason that parents must make sure that their children have qualified coaches.

A properly trained coach will know that abruptly intensifying a training regimen is likely to cause overuse injuries. Similarly, he will know that the relative hardness of the playing, running, or dancing surface is directly related to the potential for overuse injuries. For example, kneecap pain is seen when middle-distance runners move to the indoor season with little preparation for the harder pounding their legs suffer on harder, banked indoor tracks. When tennis players switch from asphalt to clay, or football players move to natural grass from astroturf, they experience less pain. When athletes move to a harder surface, their coaches must reduce their training regimen.

Properly trained coaches — and knowledgeable parents, too — will understand the importance of footwear in preventing overuse injuries of the feet, ankles, and knees. Improper footwear magnifies and accelerates overuse injuries. Well-fitting shoes with a well-contoured, firm heel counter, raised heel, and flexible forefoot are all essential for the dedicated young runner. Inadequate impact absorption material and lack of sufficient support of the heel are characteristics of poor footwear. Three characteristics — impact absorption, support, and alignment compensation — are the focus of continuing research by the major sports shoe manufacturers. Important advances in footwear design include using nylon uppers to decrease weight; flaring and raising the heel; providing rear foot stability; and, most recently, incorporating special impact-absorbing material and even air cells into the soles to lessen the force of footfall. Scientific advances in running shoe design to help decrease injury have now been applied to shoes for a great variety of other sports, including basketball, aerobic dance, tennis, and soccer. And you thought they spent all their time coming up with brighter colors!

Intensive summer sports specialty camps also put youngsters at risk of overuse injury, as when a child who plays backyard basketball or pick-up hockey an hour a day is packed off to basketball or hockey camp where he must train for six to eight hours daily. The evolution of summer camp from a two- or four-week recreational experience with camping, archery, canoeing, and art to an intensive experience in one sport has dramatically increased the incidence of overuse injuries. If you plan to send your youngster to an intensive sports camp, make sure it is staffed by qualified coaches who are aware of the potential for such injuries in children.

It doesn't help that many parents ignore warnings about overtraining and, perhaps in a well-meaning way, encourage their children to overtrain. The classic example is the proud father who takes his aspiring Little League pitcher to the park every night to "throw a few." This in the face of the well-known restriction of young pitchers to six innings a week. To please and impress dad, the youngster will throw despite the pain until he comes down with a full-blown case of Little League elbow. It will be months before this kid can return to baseball action, and surgery may be necessary. Long-term growth abnormalities are common in children with this problem. Dads should remember that there's a reason for the six-inning restriction.

While I'm all in favor of organized sports for kids, it's essential that overtraining be eliminated. Whether it's running, cycling, dance, basketball, soccer, lacrosse, or basketball, the increase in the physical workload should be *gradual*. It's important to remember that injuries aren't caused simply by too much activity, but by too-rapid increases in training activity. Once again, only when we have training curricula and certification exams for coaches will we see overuse injuries begin to decline.

The Pre-Sports Physical

Many overuse injuries in children are caused by growth-related disorders, anatomical malalignments, lack of fitness, and hidden medical problems. A physician should detect these conditions in the pre-sports physical and recommend steps to remedy or alleviate them.

As we saw earlier in this chapter the growth process, especially the adolescent growth spurt, is a major contributing factor in children's overuse injuries. Even when growth-related imbalances in strength and flexibility are not the direct cause, they may certainly exacerbate overuse syndromes. We can't stop growth, of course, but imbalances should be detected in the physical exam and, most important, exercises to both strengthen and lengthen the structures involved should be recommended. I strongly recommend decreasing the intensity of training during the growth spurt and having children do special stretching exercises to help compensate for this growth-related tightening. Parents should carefully monitor their young athletes' height and weight on a monthly basis to detect these spurts and should discuss necessary modifications in training and exercises with the physician who conducts the pre-sports physical.

Conditions that we call anatomical malalignments may be revealed during the physical. Some common examples are swayback, flat feet, knock-knees, pigeon toes, and uneven pelvis. If the physician detects swayback, for example, he may recommend a specialized exercise program and perhaps bracing to correct the condition. By contrast, some rather dramatic malalignments of the legs may actually lessen the chances of injury. For example, some of the world's best runners have pronounced bowlegs and run without any related problems.

Flat feet are often cited as a cause of overuse injury in adult athletes and are often treated with inserts (orthotics) in sports footwear. I sometimes prescribe shoe inserts for young athletes. However, the pre-sports physical may reveal that the child with flat feet also has growth-related muscle and tendon imbalances, such as tight Achilles tendons or calf muscles. Often a flexibility program to relieve this tightness will take care of the symptoms that seemed to come from the feet.

Lack of fitness, a major contributor to children's overuse injuries, should be detected in even a rudimentary pre-sports physical. As we saw in Chapter 2, American children's fitness has declined at the same time that organized sports programs involving rigorous, repetitive training regimens have increased. Poor heart-lung endurance does not result in overuse injuries, but obesity and lack of strength and flexibility certainly do. Overweight kids are predisposed to a host of acute and overuse injuries, especially slippage of the ball of the hip joint. Just the other day I performed surgery on a young basketball player whose overweight caused such a hip injury. Obesity may also precipitate stress fractures in the feet and legs because of the extra force of pounding from running and jumping.

Not only are American kids fatter than they've ever been, but they're also weaker and less flexible. Kids who watch more than twenty hours of TV per week are simply not in adequate condition to endure the stresses of repetitive microtrauma. The last thing your youngster needs during the growth process is a sedentary lifestyle that makes muscles and tendons even tighter! The strength and flexibility program in Chapter 8 should go a long way toward increasing fitness and reducing the risk of overuse injury. A conditioning program will of course enhance your children's sports performance, although this should be secondary to safeguarding their health.

Certain hidden medical problems, called associated disease states, may be brought out into the open by intense sports activity. A properly performed pre-sports physical should reveal these conditions. One of the most common is a deterioration of the ball of the hip joint, known as *Legg-Perthes disease*. Intense sports activity, especially running and jumping, may aggravate Legg-Perthes and cause such symptoms as pain in the hip and thigh, a painless limp, or a mild limp with pain on the inside of the knee. This kind of situation emphasizes the need for the pre-sports physical. Mandatory physicals would go a long way toward reducing the incidence of overuse injuries in children's sports (see Chapter 7).

A Good Conditioning Program

Most overuse injuries are aggravated by lack of strength and flexibility, caused by the growth process or a sedentary lifestyle. A conditioning program geared toward increasing strength and flexibility is a major factor in reducing the incidence of such injuries. If your youngster has to work on a specific area either because of a weakness in the area or to guard against the stresses of the sport, the physician who performs the pre-sports physical should be able to prescribe a helpful conditioning program. A general strength and flexibility program is outlined in Chapter 8.

Listening to Your Child

This isn't strictly preventive, because by the time your youngster complains of pain, it may be too late. But listening to your child may be one of the most important measures a parent can take to make sure that a mild overuse condition doesn't degenerate into a full-blown syndrome that requires surgery or puts a stop to sports for several months.

Parents and coaches must listen to their young athletes. Kids aren't malingerers. If anything, they conceal pain so they can continue playing. Often children don't want to look like wimps in front of their friends. They may also be discouraged from speaking up because of the overemphasis on winning by parents and coaches. They're scared to let the adults down. For all these reasons kids should be encouraged to speak up before it's too late. Gently explain that sports are important, but not as important as good health. Injuries that are caught early on allow children to return to participation sooner than those that are concealed and allowed to worsen, and the chances of full recovery are enhanced.

Sport-Specific Overuse Injuries

	SPINE	SHOULDER	ELBOW	HIP/PELVIS	KNEE	ANKLE/FOOT	HAND/WRIST	SHIN
Aerobics	x				x	x		x
Ballet	x			x	x	x		x
Baseball		xx	xx				x	
Basketball					x	xx		x
Bicycling	x				x			
Football	x	x		xx	xx	x		
Golf	xx	x						
Gymnastics	xx	x	x	x	x	x	xx	x
Hockey								
Ice skating	x			x	x	x		

Sport-Specific Overuse Injuries

	SPINE	SHOULDER	ELBOW	HIP/PELVIS	KNEE	ANKLE/FOOT	HAND/WRIST	SHIN
Lacrosse	x			x	x	x		
Martial arts		x	xx	x	xx			
Racquetball and squash		x	xx					
Soccer				x	xx	x		x
Tennis	x	xx	xx				x	
Track and field				x	x	x		x
Volleyball		x	x		xx	xx		

xx = higher likelihood of injury

If a child complains of a recurrent ache or pain for more than a week, you should have the problem checked immediately by a physician. However, parents should always beware of a diagnosis of "growing pains." Pain is not a natural part of growth; it's a sign of tissue injury. It is the body's early warning system, and it must be respected.

Different sports are hard on different parts of a youngster's body. Parents should know which anatomical sites are at risk of overuse injury in the specific sports their children play. For example, parents of swimmers, rowers, and baseball and tennis players should be vigilant in detecting elbow and shoulder pain in their kids; for the parents of runners and soccer players, pain in a hip, knee, or ankle should be a red flag signaling a possible overuse injury. (Consult the table on pages 122–23 for potential overuse injury sites for specific sports.)

Warning!

So far I have divided children's sports injuries into acute and overuse types. But we must be careful not to assume that all pain is sports-related. Children are subject to infections, tumors, and special diseases not experienced by adults. Two examples from my case files spring to mind.

One fifteen-year-old soccer player who complained of knee pain was evaluated by an uncertified trainer who told him the problem was runner's knee. The pain continued, and the athlete finally ended up in the sports medicine clinic at Boston's Children's Hospital. X rays and a CAT scan revealed that his knee pain was caused by a tumor of the tibia, adjacent to the knee. Needless to say, ice packs and stretching exercises didn't help his problem.

A fourteen-year-old tennis player complained of back pain and stiffness. A well-meaning coach reassured his parents that many young tennis players develop this when the intensity of their training program increases. He recommended a practitioner of massage and manipulation who "had really helped a lot of kids." The pain continued. Proper medical evaluation, with a careful physical exam, X rays, and a computerized bone scan revealed that his pain was caused by an unusual tumor, fortunately benign, an *osteoid osteoma,* seen only in children and young adults. Thankfully, surgery led to complete recovery.

These examples show that sports are not the root of all pain in all kids. Often a serious medical problem may exist. Parents should rely on a carefully chosen physician to treat their children.

6

• • • • •

Stress and
Psychological Injuries

The parents of a young dancer noticed that their daughter's teeth were gradually becoming discolored. Subsequently they discovered that peer pressure to keep her weight down had inspired the teenager to vomit after each meal. A swimming coach at a Boston area college was unable to persuade his two best freshman competitors, "burned out" from high school competition, not to drop out of the program. One young hockey player developed such a fear of competing because of his father's "win at all costs" attitude that he began refusing to show up for games. A top swimmer from New England developed "reflex sympathetic dystrophy," in which the stress of competition caused a relatively minor knee injury to progress to the stage where amputation was seriously considered.

These are all cases I've seen in the last couple of years, reflecting a growing incidence of psychological problems in child athletes, or psychological injuries, as they may be called. Contrary to what some people believe, these aren't cases of malingering. Malingering means faking a problem, and kids just don't do this. The problems we see are caused by real stress and, significantly, they are growing in number and seriousness. It's a disturbing trend and leads to the obvious question: are organized sports for kids psychologically beneficial, as once thought, or can they be damaging?

In fact, the effect of organized sports on children has traditionally been judged on the basis of the potential for emotional, not physical, damage. Even in the early 1900s the question whether youth sports programs were psychologically injurious was intensely debated by school personnel, organized athletic groups, and interested professionals, including physicians and psychologists. The explosion of youth sports programs in the last twenty years has sparked renewed and more vigorous debate. Supporters of organized sports for kids laud the building of democratic values, good citizenship, and competitive spirit, while detractors insist that the programs promote cheating, aggression, elitism, blind obedience, and psychological problems associated with competitive stress.

Critics are concerned not only with the negative effects sports have on children, but with the positive effects they *don't* have. These observers point out that in substituting organized sports for free play, something valuable has been lost. Because free play takes place away from the watchful eye — some would say meddling hand! — of adults, children are able to establish their own standards, organize themselves, and create an environment in which everyone participates. Edward Devereaux, the famed Cornell developmental psychologist, summed up these concerns in his essay, "Backyard vs. Little League Baseball." He wrote, " 'Little Leagueism' is threatening to wipe out the spontaneous culture of free play and games in American children, and is therefore robbing our children not only of their childish fun, but also of their most valuable learning experiences."

Many people have advocated dismantling the entire structure of organized children's sports. "Give sports back to the kids!" is their rallying cry. But this is highly unlikely to happen. The societal changes that changed children's sports from unstructured to organized aren't likely to be reversed. Like it or not, organized sports are here to stay.

Thankfully, we're coming to understand that sports themselves aren't harmful. Rather it is the social context in which organized children's sports take place that can be either psychologically damaging or beneficial. In a damaging environment kids may be pressured too hard to win or to perform athletic tasks they're not capable of. They may be exposed to adult behavior that teaches them that it's all right to cheat, swear, fight, and verbally abuse their opponents and game officials. Kids who remain in such programs are unlikely to benefit psychologically from their sports experience, and they may actually be harmed.

There is growing evidence that kids are dropping out of youth sports programs in unprecedented numbers because of the way the programs are run. A recent study by the National Athletic Trainers Association revealed that a full *70 percent* of high school boys drop out of all organized sports by the age of fifteen, never to return. A study recently done in the United States and Canada revealed that the main reasons children drop out of sports are:

- Not getting to play
- Abusive coaching
- An overemphasis on winning that creates stress and reduces fun
- Overorganization, excessive repetition, and regimentation, leading to boredom
- Excessive fear of failure, including frustration or failure to achieve personal or team goals
- Mismatching for physical size and maturation

In addition to those who drop out are the many who are deliberately excluded. Children as young as eight years old are cut from teams or benched permanently because of a supposed lack of ability. Kids who are excluded from a sport are unlikely to get interested in sports again. In later life they may develop feelings of inadequacy, insecurity, and inferiority because of their inability to "make it" in sports. During a conversation with the son of a nurse at Boston Children's Hospital, I discovered that he really didn't like sports. When I asked him why, he sniffed and said, "They're elitist." It turned out that as a seven-year-old, he had been cut from a soccer program in which all his friends were involved, and he had gone out of his way to avoid sports since then.

If all this reads like an indictment of organized sports, it is — and it isn't! Many youth sports programs are run with the best interests of the kids in mind, and they turn out healthy, well-adjusted players who are hooked on sports and fitness for life. I know plenty of young adults who had a safe and successful sports experience as youngsters, and as a direct result they've maintained a strong interest in sports and fitness activities.

The good news, then, is that sports are neither good nor evil. As sports commentator Louis Alley put it, sport is "a two-edged sword, capable of cutting in opposite directions. The direction the sword cuts depends on those who swing it, not on the sword itself." Clearly, with sports increasingly under adult control, it is adults who hold the two-edged sword, who make it swing for good or ill. But do adults exert too much control? What impact does organized sports have on children's personality and character development? And what is the relationship between competitive stress and injuries?

Organized Children's Sports: For Adults Only?

Critics say that adults — parents and coaches — have ruined organized sports for children. They argue that children would be far better off left alone to organize their own activities. However, it seems ludicrous to me that we should abolish organized sports for kids because "grown-ups" can't behave like adults. Can adults create a psychologically healthy environment in which all children benefit from the organized sports experience? I believe we can if we remember that children's sports are for children, not adults!

Adults become overinvolved in children's sports for all sorts of reasons. Parents regard their children as an extension of themselves, and many believe that a child's good sports performance will enhance the parents' standing in the community. It's natural for a parent to be proud of a child who performs well, whether it's in sports, academics, or social situations. Parents are usually excused for trumpeting their children's achievements to friends and neighbors — within reason. I was certainly proud of my daughters' rowing achievements. But there is a big difference between encouraging your child to participate in sports and being proud of their achievements and effort, on the one hand, and forcing them into a sport they're not interested in or pushing them too hard to be successful so that you feel good, on the other. Similarly, coaches may feel their status in the community is heightened by a championship season, and there's nothing wrong with feeling a sense of pride and accomplishment about that. But when that coach sacrifices his athletes' physical and emotional health by pushing them too hard to succeed, he's abusing his authority.

Most coaches and parents don't overstep the line that separates healthy pride from unhealthy pressure. But too many do, and unfortunately their actions may affect all the children in a program. Three of the most blatant manifestations of adult overinvolvement in children's sports are an overemphasis on winning, adult performance expectations, and inappropriate behavior at games.

The "win at all costs" mentality that pervades some youth programs is deeply troubling. Adults often confuse the pleasure children derive from sports with the desire to win. In fact, children place far more emphasis on participating than they do on winning. Any doubts on this subject have been blown away by several studies showing that kids overwhelmingly preferred to play on a losing team than to be benched all the time on a winning team. There's nothing wrong with encouraging children to play to win, but it's the effort involved in playing to win that should be celebrated, not the winning itself.

Parents and coaches tend to impose their own standards on children, to expect far too much in terms of performance and levels of commitment and involvement. Children who don't yet have the skill or coordination to perform an athletic task are sometimes harangued by a parent or coach who doesn't understand that he is looking at the game from an adult perspective. Recently I stopped to watch a children's soccer practice and saw the coach trying to teach a group of seven- to eight-year-olds to shoot at goal. These youngsters simply didn't have the requisite motor skills to kick the ball correctly most of the time, but the coach was berating them for "not trying." He expected these children to perform with the skills and strength of young men, and when they couldn't he blamed them for being lazy or nonattentive. We must remember that our kids are not as well coordinated as they will be when they're fully developed, and we shouldn't criticize their inability to perform like adults.

The behavior of adults at youth sports events has also become a cause for major concern. Many parents and coaches simply become too emotional during games and behave in a manner that may prevent children from enjoying the experience. Parents commonly boo the opponents, game officials, and even members of their own child's team. I recently heard a high school hockey player describe the "welcome" his team got when they skated onto the ice to play the high school in the next town: all the adults by the tunnel were spitting on his team! Parents and coaches have even been known to start fights with each other and with officials.

Two prominent sports scientists, Ranier Martens and Vern

Seefeldt, have come up with the following guidelines for parents attending a child's sports event:

• Remain seated in the spectator area during the contest.
• Do not yell instructions or criticisms to the children.
• Do not make derogatory comments about athletes, parents of the opposing team, officials, or league administrators.
• Do not interfere with the coach. You must relinquish the responsibility for your child to the coach during the contest.

Many adults don't realize how their behavior comes across. For example, one major study showed that coaches, when defining their goals for their athletes, overwhelmingly cited socialization and fun as the main objectives of the program and unanimously agreed that winning should not be the main emphasis. But there was a significant gap between what the coaches said and what they did. Researchers compared their answers with observations and interviews with children in the programs and found a discrepancy between the coaches' perceptions and reality. I've experienced this discrepancy firsthand. Once I confronted a coach who I thought was being terribly hard on his young players. He was indignant. "The kids love it!" he exclaimed. "And those that don't, hey, I don't need 'em."

The problem with adults getting overinvolved in children's sports is that it increases competitive stress. Many psychologists describe competitive stress as the tension between the uncertainty of the outcome of a competitive situation and the importance of the outcome. If the child is able to cope with the level of competitive stress in a particular program, she will probably enjoy the experience. But if the level of competitive stress is too high, she will dislike the program and seek ways to get out of it. By overemphasizing winning, imposing unrealistic standards, and behaving inappropriately during an event, adults magnify the importance of that event and may make the level of competitive

The Relationship Between Performance and Stress in Child Athletes

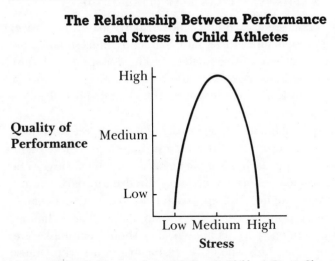

Quality of Performance

(Adapted from R. Martens, *Joy and Sadness in Children's Sports.* Champaign, Ill.: Human Kinetics, 1975)

stress too high for the child to bear. The child may decide to quit, or her athletic performance may suffer, thus intensifying the stress.

Some signs that your child is suffering from too much competitive stress are hyperactivity coupled with depression, sleep and eating disorders, rashes, nausea, headaches, muscle stiffness, lethargy, changes in academic performance, and frequent aches and pains from sports. Many parents and coaches try to "psych" up a child athlete by emphasizing the importance of the sport and of the child's performance in achieving victory. In fact, psyching up is probably the last thing adults should do to enhance a child's performance. Increasing the level of competitive stress or anxiety may be beneficial to adult athletes, whose skills are well developed. But for child athletes, whose skills are usually barely developed, anxiety can ruin performance (see the graph above).

What should adults do to shape a social context in which we

would all be happy to see our children participate? To answer this question, remember that youth sports programs should build fitness and teach good fitness habits, teach basic sports skills and healthy competition, develop self-esteem, allow children to be with their friends in a healthy environment, and above all, allow participants to have fun!

Most responsible parents and coaches would agree with these objectives, but they might differ greatly on how to achieve them. The two basic approaches are the negative and the positive. The positive approach involves motivating children to perform in a desirable way; the negative approach tries to eliminate negative traits through punishment and criticism, or the fear of failure. Without exception, parents and coaches should emphasize the positive approach. Kids who leave a game or practice with a sense of pride and satisfaction engendered by the coach on the field and by parents on the sidelines are far more likely to want to continue participating than those who feel humiliated and insecure.

Rewarding children with praise, a pat on the back, or a congratulatory smile will go a long way toward maintaining their enthusiasm. Parents and coaches should be diligent in rewarding effort, not only achievement. Of course, it's easy to cheer the player who hits a home run, sinks a basket, or scores a goal, but it's not difficult to tell which players are trying their hardest and cheer them too. Children who are rewarded with positive reinforcement are more likely to improve in skill than those who experience negative reinforcement. Those who are continually criticized build up a simple defense mechanism: they give up. That way, the next time a parent or coach questions their ability, they can say to themselves, "Well, I just wasn't trying." Adults should always encourage child athletes. The more accomplished athletes probably don't need as much encouragement as the mediocre ones, who may drop out of the program without some incentive.

Conversely, parents and coaches should strictly avoid punishment — I don't mean just running laps or doing push-ups, which can cause a child to develop a negative attitude toward sports, but also verbal insults or sarcastic comments about a player's performance. One of the most devastating experiences for a child is to come off the sports field and have a parent say, "What was *your* problem today?" Even a disappointed look from a parent or coach can make a child's heart sink. No matter whether he wins or loses, parents should always show love and encouragement. Coaches should always look for the positive in a child's performance.

Too many adults adhere to the "Vince Lombardi Motivation Theory," in which intimidation, insults, and fear of failure supposedly inspire players. This approach is still seen on television screens, with coaches belittling their players on the sidelines and in locker rooms. But don't forget, these tactics are being used on highly accomplished adult athletes. Children rarely have the confidence or self-esteem to turn harsh scolding to good effect. In fact, as we've seen, excess stress usually spoils the child's performance.

Above all, adults should remember that sports are a learning experience, and winning is not the sole objective. Children should be encouraged to learn the fundamentals of the sport, interact with other youngsters, and above all have fun. This approach almost always guarantees that the child will continue to participate.

Two controversial issues in children's sports involve benching and cutting of players. Coaches who regard winning as the most important element in children's sports are known to cut even eight-year-olds from a team. One of the first questions I ask my young patients is how they're enjoying sports. Almost nothing makes me feel so bad as when a child looks at me with a crestfallen face and tells me he was cut because he "wasn't good enough." It seems absurd that we should encourage children to try out for a team and then exclude them at the outset. Children don't need to learn these brutal lessons of life — "survival of the fittest" and so on — at this early stage. I see absolutely no reason why *any* child should be prevented from taking part in a program if he or she is healthy enough, particularly before the age of fourteen.

Similarly, benching a player for an entire game is nonsensical if the purpose of children's sports is to give all children the chance to participate. Even the least accomplished players on a team should be given the opportunity to play alongside the best ones.

One problem with children's sports is that everyone has different objectives. The coach just may want a winning team, while parents may be determined that all the children have a good time whether they win or lose, or vice versa. I am strongly in favor of a preseason meeting of parents, coaches, and even officials to discuss the goals of the program in depth. By sitting down together and examining the purpose of the program, adults should be able to realize that sports are not just about winning. Parents and coaches should also try to emphasize the satisfaction of striving for excellence. And above all, through organized sports children should learn to feel good about themselves.

Organized Sports and Psychosocial Development

Deeply rooted in American culture is a strong belief in the connection between sports participation and personal growth and development. Leadership, responsibility, courage, initiative, and cooperation — these positive qualities are all commonly ascribed to the typical athlete. Indeed, there is evidence to suggest that sports do have positive effects on psychosocial development. For example, in a comparison of child athletes with nonathletes, the athletes scored higher in positive personality traits and social acceptance than their nonathletic counterparts. Another study demonstrated that boys in Little League exhibited superior academic achievement and motor ability and were better adjusted socially and emotionally. Teachers in one survey rated athletes higher in positive personality traits, reporting that they had "more wholesome and well-integrated personalities." Other studies found positive relationships between sports participation, on the one hand, and intelligence and personality, on the other.

One benefit of sports participation is that it stimulates the child's desire to succeed in other areas. In fact, I would argue that a positive sports experience imbues children with an achievement-oriented attitude that extends to academics and social situations.

I have presented one side of what appears to be a very shiny coin. Unfortunately, the other side of the coin is not as attractive. Just as sports can inspire positive personality growth and development, exclusion from sports can do quite the opposite. Most studies focus on children who are involved with athletic programs. They don't address what happens to children who are cut from these programs or who become so unhappy that they drop out. In a study of men who in their youth had been labeled nonathletic, the participants reported feelings of inferiority and inadequacy. This clearly supports the argument that all children should be given the opportunity to participate.

Whether sports enhance children's moral development is another highly controversial issue. Learning sportsmanship, or fair play, has always been regarded as one of the main benefits of organized sports. Democracy is founded on the concept of fair play, it is argued, and without it our society would collapse. If this is true — and I question whether it is — then our democratic values are in deep trouble, because youth sports programs are one of the last places where you can expect to find examples of good sportsmanship!

In free play, children who cheated, picked fights, or otherwise spoiled the game for the rest were excluded in one way or another, and they usually ended up mending their ways. This happened because there was less emphasis on winning. Fun was the ultimate goal, and children who spoiled the fun just weren't needed or wanted.

But organized sports for children too often stress winning at all costs, and parents and coaches often overlook sportsmanship if it stands in the way of victory. Without a doubt, the behavior of professional athletes has exacerbated this situation. Through television, American society has elevated professional athletes to almost mythical proportions, and it's not surprising that children emulate these heroes. Cheating in professional sports is rarely condemned; it's considered acceptable for athletes to try to bend the rules to win. The attitude seems to be "It isn't cheating unless you get caught." Only when the player has been caught and penalized, thus jeopardizing his team's chance of winning, does he show remorse. Interviewed by the TV newsmen in the locker room after the game, the player never talks about cheating; it's always "I feel bad about letting the guys down."

Parents and coaches who teach their children to circumvent the rules in order to win are not helping them develop a sense of what's right and wrong. It is unreasonable to expect children to grow up with respect for authority, their peers, and adversaries when what happens in the sports environment is quite the opposite. Children who grow up believing it's all right to cheat, abuse, and threaten their opponents find it difficult in later life to compete without trying to pull the same tricks they learned in Little League baseball or high school football. Once again it's up to adults to establish an environment in which effort and participation are celebrated — and that means the effort and participation not only of your child and her teammates but also of their opponents.

Another traditional belief is that sports are essential for developing children's ability to cooperate. Cooperation and sportsmanship, some say, form the glue that holds our society together. However, while free play may promote cooperation (without it, free play couldn't exist), it's somewhat misguided to suggest that children learn to cooperate in most organized sports programs. To put it bluntly, in most programs children just line up and are told what to do. Some studies have demonstrated that organized sports actually undermine children's desire to cooperate. In a study of young boys in a camp setting, it was found that when competitive activities were introduced that only one group could win, the boys showed blatant feelings of rivalry and hostility.

I firmly believe that children need to learn to cooperate in order to lead happy and productive adult lives. But now that free play has been replaced by adult-dominated organized sports, how can they learn to cooperate? Putting your child into a program with a qualified coach at the helm is one solution. Good coaches know how to structure practice sessions in which the kids must interact. Another solution is to introduce more games that stress cooperation rather than competition. Unless they are very well run, these kinds of games sometimes seem overcalculated to me and rarely take into account children's instinctive urge to compete. If organized sports are too cutthroat, these "cooperation sports" seem too much like play-acting in drama class rather than sport.

Do sports programs provide a healthy environment in which children can rid themselves of natural aggression? Or do they increase levels of frustration that promote aggression and hostility? These questions, once at the heart of disagreement over the role of sports in influencing levels of aggression, now appear irrelevant. It's clear that competition itself doesn't actively promote or defuse aggressive tendencies. Instead it is the social context of sports that determines whether children exhibit excessive aggression.

Psychological Stress and Sports Injuries

Kids who are experiencing stress in sports may develop physical problems such as rashes, headaches, nausea, and muscle stiffness. They may also sustain niggling injuries and unexplained aches and pains, or what we call psychosomatic injuries. There's a tendency to dismiss psychosomatic injuries as being "all in the head," but they're not. They are experienced as real pain. Almost always, these stress-related injuries are minor and clear up as soon as the source of the stress is removed. For example, an eleven-year-old in a highly competitive soccer program with a demanding coach may complain of knee pain. She's removed from the program because of the injury, but the next day she's running around easily in the back yard. The tendency for kids to develop these psychosomatic injuries reinforces the need for qualified adult supervision so children in sports aren't overstressed.

In some instances, though, psychosomatic forces cause very real and serious problems to develop from injuries that are initially diagnosed as minor, such as sprained ankles and tendinitis of the ankle, knee, and shoulder. Despite treatment, the injuries don't improve. These patients continue to complain of severe discomfort and aren't able to return to sports. They may encounter unusual setbacks or interruptions in their rehabilitation that don't seem to fit the nature of the injury. I usually refer these youngsters for psychological evaluation, but unfortunately about a third of them don't follow through. They mistakenly think that the problem is purely physical and that we just aren't curing their ailment. These patients often drift from one physician to the next looking for the right ice pack or exercise prescription.

The sports-injured child who has prolonged or excessive pain from a relatively minor injury may be suffering from a highly complex disorder called *sympathetic reflex dystrophy* (SRD). This stress-related disorder, which was first identified in injured Civil War soldiers, eventually affects an entire limb when a small part is injured. For example, a child's entire leg may become painful even though only the knee or ankle is sprained. When our unsophisticated sympathetic nervous system associates an injury with a stressful activity, it increases blood flow to the injured area, increases the swelling, and triggers pain in the nerve endings. This process usually causes the pain to spread throughout the limb and well beyond the area of initial injury. Remember, this isn't an imaginary ailment; the injury actually worsens and spreads.

Until very recently, SRD was almost unheard of in children, but it's becoming increasingly prevalent, mostly in elite child athletes. The emergence of this disorder seems to be tied to the rise of organized children's sports. I almost always refer such patients for psychological evaluation. Usually a familiar pattern emerges during the initial interview. Children who develop SRD are often being pushed too hard by parents or a coach; they sometimes claim they "live for the sport," and yet they can't actually describe what they enjoy about the sport; they may reveal that their self-esteem is closely linked to sports participation; and they often have very few interests outside the sport.

Probably the best way to illustrate how this complex disorder manifests itself is through a case study. "Tim" was a fourteen-year-old elite junior tennis player who sustained a sprained left ankle. At a nearby community hospital X rays initially revealed that Tim had a mild to moderate sprain. He was immobilized and told to gradually increase his activity, a typical rehabilitation program for an injury of this kind. However, instead of a decrease in symptoms and swelling and increased ankle mobility, Tim's pain began to worsen. He described it as a burning sensation. Not only was his ankle painful, but the pain began spreading into the foot and up into the rest of the leg. By the time I saw Tim, six weeks after the injury occurred, he could barely exert any pressure on the toes of the affected limb and had to use crutches to get around. He had also developed a noticeable swelling in the foot.

My initial evaluation of Tim suggested that what was happening in his foot and ankle went well beyond what would be expected of a straightforward sprained ankle. It occurred to me almost immediately that Tim might be suffering from sympathetic reflex dystrophy. My diagnosis was confirmed by a bone scan which showed a dark area where the SRD had set in.

Tim was immediately referred to the pain service clinic at Children's Hospital where my pain specialist colleagues agreed with my diagnosis. Tim's treatment began with slow, gentle aquatic physical therapy. He was also started on nerve stimulation, an electrical technique that helps reverse nerve problems if they are caught early enough. Tim was also put on medication to reduce the irritability of the nerve injury.

Despite these early measures, Tim didn't respond and ultimately required an intermittent program of nerve blocks to help reverse this process. I have found that psychological factors usually play a large part in SRD in children, so I referred Tim to a clinical psychologist with expertise in this kind of psychosomatic illness in children. She determined that very profound psychological pressures existed in Tim's family setting. He was the only child of highly motivated and competitive parents. His father, who described himself as a self-made man, was an aggressive, hard-working, and highly successful businessman. He had worked his way through undergraduate and graduate programs in a variety of odd jobs. Tim's father had developed an interest in sports activities and had been the motivator for his son's decision to take up tennis. It appeared that his interest in Tim's tennis playing was motivated not only by a love of sports but also by social interests. He felt Tim could advance socially through his interest in tennis.

While Tim said he enjoyed tennis and enjoyed being state

champion in his age group, he also admitted that the intensive program his parents encouraged him to undertake — practice four nights a week and annual summer camps — meant he had little time to spend with friends, and he felt he had very few friends left. Indeed, Tim was apparently regarded as a loner or oddball at school. His sense of isolation was compounded by his parents' decision to send him off to a private school. In his neighborhood and community he was referred to as a snob.

Although Tim's mother showed a vague interest in her son's success, she was more preoccupied with her career than her son's tennis involvement. Because her professional life was so time-consuming, she was able to devote little time to his social development. Tim seemed emotionally distant from his mother and admitted he wouldn't consider going to her with a problem. The psychologist's conclusion was that this was a family ridden with tension and anger, particularly Tim's anger at his parents because of their insistence that he give up a normal childhood for tennis. In turn, Tim's parents had developed subconscious feelings of anger toward Tim because of his injury, which was inconveniencing them and also preventing him from competing in the sport they had chosen for him.

Through a combination of medical intervention, specific physical therapy, and techniques to alleviate and reverse this neurological process, as well as very specific psychological counseling for Tim and the family, Tim did recover from this injury. However, he was unable to resume playing high-level tennis for approximately nine months. But he decided on his own to return to the sport. He became a skilled and accomplished tennis player and represented his college as a freshman.

Participation in sports involves a complex interaction of physical, psychological, and social factors. Some children cope easily with the stress of competition, and their participation leads to enhanced self-esteem and personal growth; others cope poorly, and not only are they likely to suffer psychosocial problems, but they're also more likely to sustain injuries, some of them serious. Clearly, psychotherapeutic intervention may be necessary in those cases where organized sports cause a child emotional stress.

But it is we adults who determine the all-important social context in which sports take place, and I would like to think that it is possible to dramatically reduce the incidence of psychological problems among child athletes by making the American sports experience a positive one, from which all children can benefit.

7

• • • • •

The Pre-Sports Physical as Preventive Medicine

Last year a Boston-area high school basketball player collapsed and died during a game because of an undiagnosed heart condition. Waiting for me right now in my clinic is a young gymnast with severe back pain due to tight muscles and ligaments. What do these two cases have in common? Answer: both might have been avoided had each child undergone a proper pre-sports physical (known in medical circles as a preparticipation medical evaluation).

According to the American Medical Association, every child athlete should have a "thorough preseason history and medical evaluation." Why is this so important? Put simply, such an evaluation can detect conditions that may predispose a child to injury and can provide treatment to alleviate these problems.

These are the main goals of your child's pre-sports checkup:

- To assess overall health.
- To detect conditions that might cause injury.
- To detect conditions that disqualify a child from participation in certain sports.
- To assess fitness for the chosen sport.
- To determine maturity as a help in sports counseling.

A thorough physical is especially important if your child is just beginning sports. At this stage she is a "blank slate." As she becomes more experienced as an athlete, significant medical problems are less likely to be revealed during subsequent checkups. The physician will be more concerned with examining the residuals of previous injuries than with inherent problems. Also initial examination may reveal a particular condition for the first time. Scoliosis, heart murmurs, a single testicle, and knee instability are all examples of common medical conditions that are first detected during the pre-sports physical. It is vital that the physician have a record of the nature and severity of such conditions before the child begins in sports.

Unfortunately, far too many adults involved in youth sports — parents, coaches, even team physicians — have a "penny-wise" attitude toward this evaluation. I see hundreds of parents every year who recognize its importance only after it's too late, when they're sitting in the sports clinic beside one very miserable youngster! Many of the injuries I see could have been prevented if the children had had a good physical. And that goes for hundreds of thousands of sports-injured kids every year.

You might ask why there's suddenly a need for these sports exams. The main reason is that the physical and psychological demands of children's sports have increased dramatically since the olden days of sandlot sports and free play. These increased demands and the corresponding increase in the rate and severity of children's sports injuries emphasize that the pre-sports physical should be the cornerstone of sports care for young athletes. But this ideal is light years away from reality in most cases. As the American Academy of Pediatrics recently stated, the pre-sports physical is often "superficial, hurried, and frequently designed to fulfill legal requirements — the antithesis of good medical care." I've heard of an entire football team, forty-five kids in all, examined by a single physician in just three quarters of an hour. All he did was walk up and down the line, saying,

"Open your mouth, bend forward, bend backward, okay you're fine."

I feel so strongly about the role of the pre-sports physical that in 1986 I initiated the Children's Hospital Athletic Medical Preventive Screening program, known as CHAMPS. At the CHAMPS clinic my staff and I perform an intensive battery of painless tests to measure body composition, strength and endurance, and maturity. Using the information from these tests, we develop a personalized exercise program to correct children's weaknesses and build on their strengths. For example, I often see boys and girls with swayback brought on by the growth process and often exacerbated by a sedentary lifestyle. To correct the swayback and avoid the danger of overuse sports injuries, I put the child on a carefully structured program of strength and flexibility training.

Some kids who come into CHAMPS are the stars of their team, and certainly their motor skills and coordination are well developed. But when they're put through their paces in the cardiovascular endurance tests I find they can barely make it around a 400-meter track! The parents of these kids have been fooled into thinking their kids are fit because they can bat a ball or sink a basketball with ease. As we saw in Chapter 3, motor skills and health fitness are two very different things. It's great to have motor skills, but health fitness is far more important for preventing degenerative diseases in later life. At the CHAMPS program we're able to differentiate between these two and provide an exercise regimen to remedy deficiencies in health fitness.

Back to reality, folks. The fact is that most parents, and that probably includes you, of sports-active kids don't have access to a CHAMPS-type program. But this doesn't mean you have to settle for the outdated locker room lineup. What are the options available to parents who want their child to have a good physical exam?

I strongly suggest, for several reasons, that your child's examination be performed by your primary care physician (pediatrician or family physician). Continuity is one obvious advantage. Your primary care physician has ready access to your child's medical history, as well as familiarity with any emotional problems and recurring illnesses or injuries. He or she probably has an insight into your relationship with your child, which will assist in any counseling that is necessary. On a practical level the primary care physician is equipped to provide ongoing treatment and rehabilitation.

However, having the primary care physician perform the pre-sports physical does have certain drawbacks. The most obvious one is that your physician may not be familiar with sports medicine. Despite the rise in organized sports and the health importance of fitness and exercise, few medical schools include sports medicine in their curricula. But as the explosion in organized sports showers family physicians with sports medicine–related questions, patients with sports injuries, and requests for sports-care health services, more physicians are pursuing postgraduate education in this field. At some point in their careers most physicians have a brush with sports medicine as an adviser to parents, a part-time team physician, or simply as the parent of a child athlete. Programs such as the Team Physician Curriculum of the American College of Sports Medicine, created in 1988, should do much to answer the need for expertise in this area.

But what should you do if you discover that your primary care physician has absolutely no knowledge of sports medicine? Unfortunately, like the old dog in the proverb, some physicians don't want to learn any new tricks. In that case the physical should be done by a physician who is familiar with the demands of sports. Today many communities, even small towns, have sports medicine clinics. However, you should be absolutely sure that the clinic is staffed by fully licensed physicians. And the clinic's report should be sent to your primary care physician to maintain that basic continuity.

Opinions vary as to the timing of the pre-sports checkup. I feel strongly that it should take place three to four months before the sports season starts. This allows plenty of time for the physician to evaluate and correct any specific problems rather than having to improvise a remedial program at the last minute. For example, the knee disorder called Osgood-Schlatter's disease needs at least three months to be corrected, but many kids with this condition come to see me just a couple of weeks before the season begins. Try telling a soccer-mad youngster that he has to miss the first half of the season while he does leg-lifting exercises!

The emphasis in the pre-sports physical should be on quality, not quantity. Once a year is ideal. To have an examination before each season is time-consuming as well as expensive. And there's little to be gained from such frequent exams. Your family physician's records of injuries, illnesses, and medical care will indicate if your child needs medical attention before the next sport begins. For example, if your child has a history of tendinitis, the physician should check for any residuals of this condition and should prescribe stretching exercises to reduce the risk of its recurrence. However, if your child is starting a sports program radically different from the one she is used to, let's say she's going to switch from basketball to gymnastics, then a sport-specific physical should be done to ensure she's fit to participate in that program.

To be deemed healthy, a child should have at least basal levels of cardiovascular, nutritional, and musculoskeletal fitness. A youngster who plans to join even a moderately intensive sports program may need to be more fit in particular areas specific to the sport. The examining physician should determine whether your child is fit for the sport he is going to play. The American Academy of Pediatrics recently stated that the pre-sports physical should be sport-specific. For example, if your child is starting a gymnastics program, particular attention should be paid to the elbows, wrists, back, pelvis, and knees; a baseball player's throwing arm should be given special attention.

All the components of the physical, including the assessment of body composition, cardiovascular fitness, strength and flexibility, and diet, are important, but I've come to believe that the most important components are the medical history and the physical examination.

Medical history. This is extremely important because it alerts the examining physician to previous illnesses, injuries, and operations that may have significant bearing on the child's fitness for athletics. Well over half of the problems I encounter in child athletes are identified in the history. A common example of a serious but hidden injury that the medical history can reveal is an undiagnosed fracture of the carpal navicular bone in the wrist. Your child may dismiss the wrist pain as a sprain. "It's no big deal, Mom," he says, and you and dad have no reason to suspect otherwise. But, in fact, if a carpal navicular bone fracture is undiagnosed, it can have serious arthritic consequences for your child in later life. Because of the importance of the medical history, you should assist your child in completing the answers *accurately*. One study showed that without parental input, only one third of children completed their medical histories accurately.

Some of the areas to remember when helping your child fill out the history include:

- Hospitalizations and surgery
- Medications
- Allergies
- Tetanus immunization status
- Family cardiovascular problems
- Skin problems
- Sprains, strains, and fractures
- Problems coping with heat or cold

Physical examination. A great deal has been written about the cardiovascular component of the physical examination. If your child does not have good cardiovascular endurance, fatigue-related injuries like sprained ankles and twisted knees are more likely to occur. However, I feel that insufficient attention is paid to assessing the strength of muscles and bones and the flexibility of muscles, ligaments, and joints. In my experience most children's sports injuries result from problems of the musculoskeletal system. The physical should include an examination for joint function, range of motion, and areas of pain. Clearly, restricted range of motion in joints, tight muscles, and lack of muscle strength will create problems for the young athlete. The risk of injury increases when there is less flexibility. During dynamic activity, suddenly stretching a tight-ligamented joint such as a knee or ankle or the tight muscles crossing that joint may result in injury to the joint or muscle. Special emphasis should be given to ankles and knees because of the high incidence of injury to those areas. If your child displays a lack of flexibility, she should begin a program of strength and flexibility training before the sports season begins. The examining physician can give you exercise to overcome particular problems, or you can follow my exercise program in the next chapter.

After the physical, you and your child should discuss the results with the examining physician. Be sure to find out about any conditions that have to be corrected or rehabilitated before your youngster can begin sports participation. After reviewing the history and physical examination, the physician has several choices:

- Allow full, unlimited participation.
- Withhold clearance until a problem is corrected.
- Withhold clearance until additional examinations are performed.
- Allow participation in certain sports.
- Not allow participation.

The physician's decision is usually based on the American Academy of Pediatrics' well-established "Recommendations for

Disqualifying Conditions for Sports Participation

●

CONDITIONS	COLLI-SION*	CONTACT†	NON-CONTACT‡	OTHER§
General				
Acute infections: Respiratory, genitourinary, infectious mononucleosis, hepatitis, active rheumatic fever, active tuberculosis	x	x	x	x
Obvious physical immaturity in comparison with other competitors	x	x		
Hemorrhagic disease: Hemophilia, purpura, and other serious bleeding tendencies	x	x	x	
Diabetes, inadequately controlled	x	x	x	x
Diabetes, controlled	††	††	††	††
Jaundice	x	x	x	x
Eyes				
Absence or loss of function of one eye	x	x		
Respiratory				
Tuberculosis (active or symptomatic)	x	x	x	x
Severe pulmonary insufficiency	x	x	x	x

Disqualifying Conditions for Sports Participation

●

CONDITIONS	COLLI-SION*	CONTACT†	NON-CONTACT‡	OTHER§
Cardiovascular				
Mitral stenosis, aortic stenosis, aortic insufficiency, coarctation of aorta, cyanotic heart disease, recent carditis of any etiology	x	x	x	x
Hypertension on organic basis	x	x	x	x
Previous heart surgery for congenital or acquired heart disease	‖	‖	‖	‖
Liver, enlarged	x	x		
Skin				
Boils, impetigo, and herpes simplex gladiatorum	x	x		
Spleen, enlarged	x	x		
Hernia				
Inguinal or femoral hernia	x	x	x	
Musculoskeletal				
Symptomatic abnormalities of inflammations	x	x	x	x
Functional inadequacy of the musculoskeletal system, congenital or acquired, incompatible with the contact or skill demands of the sport	x	x	x	

Disqualifying Conditions for Sports Participation

●

CONDITIONS	COLLI-SION*	CONTACT†	NON-CONTACT‡	OTHER§
Neurologic				
History or symptoms of previous serious head trauma or repeated concussions	x			
Controlled convulsive disorder	¶	¶	¶	¶
Convulsive disorder not moderately well controlled by medication	x			
Previous surgery on head	x	x		
Renal				
Absence of one kidney	x	x		
Renal disease	x	x	x	x
Genitalia				
Absence of one testicle	**	**	**	**
Undescended testicle	**	**	**	**

*Football, rugby, hockey, lacrosse, and so forth.
†Baseball, soccer, basketball, wrestling, and so forth.
‡Cross country, track, tennis, crew, swimming, and so forth.
§Bowling, gulf, archery, field events, and so forth.
††No exclusions.
‖Each patient should be judged on an individual basis in conjunction with his cardiologist and surgeon.
¶Each patient should be judged on an individual basis. All things being equal, it is probably better to encourage a young boy or girl to participate in a noncontact sport rather than a contact sport. However, if a patient has a desire to play a contact sport and this is deemed a major ameliorating factor in his or her adjustment to school, associates, and the seizure disorder, serious consideration should be given to letting him or her participate if the seizures are moderately well controlled or the patient is under good medical management.
**The committee approves the concept of contact sports participation for youths with only one testicle or with an undescended testicle(s), except in specific instances such as an inguinal canal undescended testicle(s), following appropriate medical evauation to rule out unusual injury risk. However, the athlete, parents, and school authorities should be fully

Participation in Competitive Sports." These guidelines list medical conditions that disqualify children from participation in collision, contact, and noncontact sports (see the table on pages 152–54). For example, a child with an enlarged liver shouldn't be allowed to play a contact or collision sport like football, but may participate in non-contact sports such as tennis and track. Thanks to the great advances in modern medicine and the ever-expanding scope of available sports, the vast majority of youngsters, regardless of illness or disability, have the potential to participate in some sport. For much more on the sports opportunities for children with a disability or chronic illness, see Chapters 11 and 12.

informed that participation in contact sports for youths with only one testicle carries a slight injury risk to the remaining healthy testicle. Fertility may be adversely affected following an injury. But the chances of an injury to a descended testicle are rare, and the injury risk can be further substantially minimized with an athletic supporter and protective device.

Reprinted by permission of the American Academy of Pediatrics.

8

•••••

Strength and Flexibility:
Keys to Preventing Injuries

All three components of health fitness: heart-lung endurance (cardiovascular), ratio of fat to lean muscle (nutritional), and strength and flexibility (musculoskeletal) are vital for lifetime good health. On the whole, cardiovascular and nutritional fitness have received the most attention. That's understandable: improving these components of health fitness is tied closely to reducing the frightening levels of cardiovascular disease in this country. It hasn't done the cause any harm that aerobic exercise, which is the best way to achieve cardiovascular and nutritional fitness, may also help make us slimmer! But it concerns me that strength and flexibility haven't received sufficient attention. True, these elements don't contribute to reducing the risk of life-threatening diseases, but they make an enormous difference to medical conditions that affect our quality of life. Two conditions that are closely tied to declining strength and flexibility are osteoporosis and back pain. After twenty years of treating sports injuries I'm also convinced that strength and flexibility are *more* important than cardiovascular and nutritional fitness in preventing both acute and overuse sports injuries.

Part of the reason that strength training hasn't been given the attention it deserves is that many people automatically associate it with "body building" — all those oiled, rippling torsos in teeny-weeny bikinis. That kind of conditioning has nothing to do with the strength and flexibility training that I advocate for child athletes.

The Decline of Strength and Flexibility

We know that strength and flexibility are essential for daily living and injury prevention, but all the evidence suggests that our children's levels of these factors are sinking miserably. How's this for a scary glimpse?

- 70 percent of boys and girls can't do a single chin-up.
- 40 percent of boys and 70 percent of girls can do only one push-up.
- 40 percent of boys can't touch their toes.
- 25 percent of all kids can't do one proper sit-up.

Pretty pathetic, isn't it? As we saw in Chapter 2, children's increasingly sedentary lives — too much TV, not enough P.E. — contribute to obesity, poor heart and lung endurance, and low strength and flexibility. Kids who watch more than twenty hours of television a week simply aren't giving their muscles the workout they need. At the same time, all those hours spent curled up on the couch watching TV or scrunched in front of a computer game screen are causing their muscles and joints to tighten up. Our bodies were designed to be used, and when they're not being used, they don't work very well. Our bodies work better the more they're used.

The Benefits of Strength and Flexibility

If our muscles and bones aren't functioning efficiently, how can we call ourselves healthy, let alone fit? Strength and flexibility allow us to enjoy life more because all our movements are more comfortable, from taking out the trash to reaching around to the back seat of the station wagon to wipe ice cream off a child's face. These important elements also help us in emergency situations. Listen to what the American Alliance of Health, Physical Education, Recreation, and Dance (AAHPERD) says: "In an emergency, the ability to apply force with the upper body can mean the difference between serious injury and escaping harm."

If all this doesn't convince you that strength and flexibility are important, just consider that the rising incidence of lower-back pain — the number-one reason for workers' compensation claims — has been tied to declining strength and flexibility. Lower-back pain is usually caused by weak abdominal muscles and tight back muscles. If these two conditions begin in childhood, you are virtually guaranteed a life of lower-back pain. It has also been proven that strengthening the bones in childhood and adolescence reduces the risk of osteoporosis.

In sports the benefits of strength and flexibility are very clear:

- Improved performance
- Reduced risk of injury
- Fewer aches and pains after playing

Improved performance is a welcome result of strength and flexibility training. Flexibility makes kids quicker and more agile, which is useful in all sports, even those that don't depend on body-bending movements. Baseball and basketball players benefit from an all-around flexibility program. Specialized flexibility programs are essential for conditioning dancers and gymnasts.

The positive effects of strength training have been well demonstrated in adolescents of both sexes in sports as varied as distance running, football, and gymnastics. Strength training is particularly useful in sports requiring controlled or explosive running, jumping, throwing, pushing, and pulling.

But much more important in my view is the role strength and flexibility play in preventing injury. Many of the skills we associate with gymnastics, figure skating, and wrestling require extra flexibility of certain muscles and joints. If an athlete tries to perform these maneuvers without the necessary range of motion in muscles and joints, an injury will probably occur. Even the seemingly benign twists and turns of soccer can cause injury in a "tight" athlete. Increasing the range of motion will minimize the chance of a tear-type injury.

Strengthening muscles enables us to resist sprains and strains. Strong muscle tissue is also better able to withstand the normal trauma of contact and collision sports such as football, soccer, basketball, and hockey by providing greater protection to internal structures. Strong muscles also lessen the jarring impact in running and jumping. It's not well recognized that exercise also enlarges and strengthens our bones. Just look at a tennis player's playing arm. The muscles are more developed than in the opposite arm, and so are the bones. If you put your fingers around the wrists of both arms, you'll find that the bones of the playing arm are bigger. Not surprisingly, strong bones are a boon in later life, when bones tend to become weak and brittle.

All of us — children, parents, and grandparents — can benefit from a strength and flexibility program. But it is especially important for children because of their tendency to develop tight muscles, ligaments, and tendons during the growth process. As we learned in Chapter 4, children's bones grow first, so during the growth spurt, the soft tissues — muscles, ligaments, and tendons — tend to get tighter and to be vulnerable to injury. The growth process also causes imbalances in muscle strength and flexibility, which can be remedied by a strength training program. When your child has her pre-sports physical, find out what exercises she should do to remedy tightness or strength imbalances.

Flexibility Training

Children should do flexibility exercises daily to increase their range of motion. You should know how to lead your kids in a flexibility program, which is good for adults, too! Not only that, but it makes you feel great. Tie the stretching exercises in with family fitness activities: a brisk walk or slow jog to the park, followed by a period of stretching and calisthenics, then a game of soccer or frisbee is a wonderful way to spend a couple of hours with your children. It also involves all three components of health fitness — cardiovascular, nutritional, and musculoskeletal. Don't underestimate your children and assume that they will resist your efforts to get them started on a flexibility program. Explain the benefits of flexibility to them directly to enlist their cooperation.

In addition, kids should be taught the relationship between flexibility and sports performance. A good coach should be able to convey the importance of stretching exercises. A trained soccer coach will know that the groin strains suffered by many soccer players, both young and old, can be avoided through simple exercises for the groin area. Gymnastics coaches are aware that the incidence of back injuries can be reduced by stretching out the back muscles. Of course, this indicates once again the need for trained coaches.

Flexibility exercises should be done both before and after sports. All sports activities should have five stages:

WARM-UP — STRETCH — SPORTS ACTIVITY —
COOL-DOWN — STRETCH

Although the principle is now well established in sports circles, many people are still unaware that the stretch should not come first. Before doing flexibility exercises, athletes should warm up their muscles by doing a gentle, repetitive activity such as fast walking, jogging, gentle bike riding, stroking around the ice, or something similar. This activity assists the stretching phase by increasing the blood flow to muscles, ligaments, and tendons and making them more pliable. You'll understand this process if you try to touch your toes now, then try again after a ten-minute jog. You'll find it's much easier after your muscles are warmed up.

After the initial warm-up comes the stretching phase. You should include at least one stretch for each of the major joint-muscle areas, including the shoulders, elbows, wrists, trunk, lower back, hips, knees, and ankles, as well as the hamstring and quadriceps muscles. After the sports activity the athlete should do a cool-down activity to let the heart rate return to normal. The final stage is stretching exercises to prevent many of the aches and pains that occur when you stop too suddenly. Both the warm-up–then–stretch and the cool-down–then–stretch should last between fifteen and twenty minutes.

Ways of Stretching

Stretching exercises have both short-term and long-term benefits. In the short term stretching increases the joints' range of motion, improves the ease of muscles crossing the joints, and increases the blood supply to soft tissues. These immediate changes, which enhance performance and help prevent injury, by themselves justify the need for stretching before exercise. Long-term benefits include enhanced comfort and better functioning of the whole system.

There are three types of stretching techniques:

- Passive: stretching to a given position and holding it.
- Active: stretching the muscle by bouncing (sometimes called ballistic stretching).
- Proprioceptive Neuromuscular Facilitation (PNF): before stretching a muscle, tensing its opposite muscle to relax the muscle that is to be stretched.

The passive technique is the one I recommend for most people, especially kids. True, improvements in flexibility have been shown with the active and PNF techniques, but each method has its problems. Active stretching uses the momentum of bouncing, by bending over and bouncing to touch your toes, for example, to stretch the hamstring muscle farther. But in using momentum, the athlete loses the control needed to stretch the muscle without stimulating the "stretch reflex." This reflex happens when the muscle feels itself stretching too far too fast and instinctively shortens, thus defeating the whole purpose of the stretch. Also muscle tissue is more likely to be damaged when it is lengthened sharply instead of gradually. For these reasons I strongly discourage both kids and adults from using the active technique. As for PNF, this is an excellent way to stretch, but it requires professional instruction and supervision and is too confusing for most kids, as well as many adults.

Frequency, Intensity, and Duration

Whether flexibility training succeeds in improving fitness depends on three factors: how often you do it (frequency), how hard you do it (intensity), and how long you do it (duration). This goes for cardiovascular as well as musculoskeletal fitness. To develop flexibility, children should do stretching exercises daily. If the pre-sports physical has revealed a severe limitation in a particular area (the hamstrings, for example), exercises should be done twice a day.

Intensity in a flexibility program refers to how much the muscles stretch during each exercise. There are several theories on intensity. The best known is the "no pain, no gain" school of thought, which holds that the muscle should be stretched until it hurts. However, this decreases the duration of the stretch, increases the chance of prompting the stretch reflex, and may cause a muscle strain. Instead of pushing muscles to the point where they hurt, children should stretch just until they feel the point of tension, known as the "action point." By not overstretching the muscle, athletes can relax while they are stretching and thus hold each position longer.

The amount of time a stretch should be held (duration) varies tremendously according to whom you ask. I recommend that exercises be held at the action point for a minimum of sixty seconds. This is probably longer than any stretch you've heard of, but our research has shown that it takes about twenty to forty seconds for the child's muscles to relax. By holding the stretch for sixty seconds, we are ensuring that the tight muscles, tendons, and ligaments are being stretched slowly, with a minimal chance of injury.

Stretching Exercises

What follows is a series of flexibility exercises that can be done independently at home or in conjunction with a sports program. The recommended length of time to hold each stretch is given. If your child is unable to hold a position for the specified time because he gets tired, that's all right. He can rest for a moment, or, where appropriate, switch to the other limb. Your child should perform the stretch as many times as is necessary to reach the recommended duration. All-around flexibility should be every-

Sport-Specific Flexibility Conditioning

	NECK	SHOULDER	LOWER BACK/TRUNK	GROIN	QUADRICEPS	HAMSTRINGS	CALF
Aerobics			X	X	X	X	X
Ballet			XX	X	X	XX	XX
Baseball	X	X	X	X		X	
Basketball		X	X	X	X	XX	XX
Bicycling	X	X			X	XX	X
Football			X	X	X	X	X
Golf			X	X			
Gymnastics	X	X	X	X	X	X	X
Hockey			X	XX	X	X	
Ice skating			X	X	X	X	X

Sport-Specific Flexibility Conditioning

	NECK	SHOULDER	LOWER BACK/TRUNK	GROIN	QUADRICEPS	HAMSTRINGS	CALF
Lacrosse	X	X	X	X	XX	XX	XX
Martial arts	X	X	X	XX	XX	XX	XX
Racquetball/squash	X	X	X	X	X	XX	XX
Soccer			X	XX	XX	XX	X
Tennis	X	X	X	X	X	X	X
Track and field			X	X	X	XX	XX
Volleyball	X	X	XX	X	XX	XX	X

xx = special emphasis

one's goal, but some sports require extra flexibility in certain areas (see the table on pages 164–65).

Remember the old saw: "If something's worth doing, it's worth doing well." This applies perfectly to flexibility and strength training. Many kids get frustrated with flexibility programs because they don't see themselves making gains. The problem is poor technique. There are no short cuts to achieving good flexibility; by trying to take short cuts children will not improve their flexibility and may even injure themselves in the process. It's important to pay close attention to technique and to the length of time you should be holding the stretch. Remember not to bounce or overstretch. Kids — and adults too — often overstretch because they're impatient to get it over with. One way to overcome this tendency is to keep yourself and your kids occupied during the stretch. Listening to relaxing music and talking can set the tone for leisurely stretching. You don't need to be uncomfortable while you're stretching. Buy a good exercise mat for yourself and each child to make yourselves more comfortable and to reinforce the importance of the activity. Finally, you should not feel any pain during a stretch. If you do, you're overstretching your muscles and should reduce the length of the stretch.

The lying full-body stretch (*relaxation*). Start by lying on your back with arms and legs outstretched. Close your eyes, relax your entire body, and inhale deeply. Hold for a count of one, then slowly exhale completely. Repeat fifteen times.

The seated neck circle (*neck*). Sit on the floor with your legs crossed Indian-style. Turn your head to the right and try to look over your right shoulder. Then slowly rotate your head to the left and look over your left shoulder. With your head facing forward, bend your neck to the right so your right ear is toward your right shoulder. Do the same thing to the left. Return your head to the center position. Bend your neck forward so your chin moves toward your chest. Then extend your neck so you're looking at the ceiling. Hold each position for thirty seconds. Be sure not to twist or jerk the neck.

Shoulder stretch (*shoulder*). Stand with your feet shoulder width apart, then raise your right arm so it's pointing straight up. Drape your right arm over the top of your head. With your left arm pull your right elbow behind your head until you feel a slight stretch in your shoulder and triceps. To maximize the effectiveness of the stretch, try not to let your head bend forward too far. Repeat the stretch on your left shoulder. Hold each side for sixty seconds.

Shoulder and side stretch (*trunk*). Stand with your right arm raised. Grasp your right elbow with your left hand behind your head and gently pull your right arm to your ear. Bend your trunk to the left until you feel a stretch in your right upper back and trunk. Hold for sixty seconds, then repeat on your right side.

Lunge (*front of the hip*). Begin with the feet together, hands on your hips, and eyes focused straight ahead. With your right foot take a big step forward. Your front foot should face straight ahead. Your back foot should also face forward, but the heel should be off the ground. Keep your shoulders back, your hips straight, and your eyes forward. Bend your forward knee, moving your pelvis forward toward the floor until you feel the action point. You should feel this stretch in the quadriceps of your back leg and in the front of that hip. Hold the stretch on each side for sixty seconds.

Standing ballet stretch (*quadriceps*). Stand on your left leg. With your left arm balance yourself, using a chair or wall. Bend your right leg back and pull your right ankle up toward your right buttock. With your right hand, pull up on your ankle so that your knee points down until you feel the action point. Hold for sixty seconds and then change sides.

Lying quadriceps and iliotibial band stretch (*front and outside of thigh*). Lie on your left side with your left knee bent at ninety degrees and your right leg straight. Then bend your right leg and grasp that ankle with your right hand. Gently pull your right heel toward your buttocks. When you feel the stretch in your right quadriceps, lower your knee toward the floor in back of your left knee. Hold for sixty seconds. This will produce a stretch in the muscles around the hip (the tensor fascia lata and the iliotibial band) as well as in the quadriceps. Repeat on the other leg.

Wall split (hamstrings and groin). To stretch both hamstrings, the lower back, and hip adductors, begin by lying beside a wall. Bend your knees, then swing around so your body is at right angles to the wall. Raise both legs so that your buttocks are flat against the wall, your legs are pointing up, and your feet are resting against the wall. Straighten the knees to stretch the hamstring and calf muscles. Then, while keeping your knees straight, gently slide your legs apart and allow gravity to pull your feet toward the floor. Continue to let your feet slide down the wall until you feel a stretch on the inner thigh. Hold each position for sixty seconds.

Posterior pelvic tilt (lower back). With the increased incidence of swayback in young athletes, particularly gymnasts, dancers, and figure skaters, this exercise is good to include in daily training. Begin by lying on your back with your legs outstretched and your hands at your sides. Gently tense your abdominal muscles and try to push them toward the floor. Simultaneously tense your buttocks and press your lower back downward toward the floor. Hold this position for six sets of ten seconds.

Seated piked hamstring stretch (hamstrings). Sit on the floor with your legs outstretched, ankles together, and toes pointed upward. Place your hands on the floor by the thighs. Look straight ahead and gently slide your hands forward. Keep your back and knees straight and try to bring your chest as close to your knees and thighs as possible. When you feel a stretch behind your knees and thighs, stop and hold this position for sixty seconds.

Wall calf stretch (calves). Stand with the feet shoulder width apart and arm's length away from a wall, post, or chair you can lean on for balance. Slowly slide your right foot directly back approximately two feet, keeping your right leg fully extended and your foot pointed slightly inward. The heels of both feet should stay flat on the floor. Look directly forward, and keep your hips and shoulders squared. Bend your left knee and slowly move your pelvis forward. Stop and hold the position for sixty seconds when you feel a stretch in your right Achilles tendon. Switch legs and repeat the exercise.

This exercise can also be performed by standing with the feet shoulder width apart and slightly turned in. Leaning against a wall with outstretched hands, allow your body to fall forward toward the wall. While keeping your back and knees straight, move your chest and hips toward the wall until you feel a stretch in the upper calf area. Hold this position for sixty seconds. As you become more flexible, you can stand farther from the wall.

The second part of this exercise stretches the entire calf muscle. Start with the feet shoulder width apart and arm's length from a wall. Slide your right foot directly back about a foot and a half. While keeping the heels of both feet flat on the ground, gently bend both knees until you feel a stretch in the calf and Achilles tendon of your back leg. Hold this position for sixty seconds and repeat for the left leg.

Toe circles (*ankles*). Sit with your knees fully straightened, your toes pointing up, and your ankles twelve inches apart. Relax your thigh and leg muscles. Begin by pointing your toes away from you. Rotate your feet away from each other in a circular motion. Make the largest circles you can. Perform fifteen circles in this direction, then do fifteen in the other direction. Repeat the exercise with your feet pointed back toward your knees.

Strength Training

For years strength training was shunned by many amateur and professional athletes. People were under the false impression that developing muscle strength with weights would make them muscle-bound and decrease the range of motion of the joints. Rubbish! Properly performed strength training doesn't *decrease* a joint's range of motion, but actually can *increase* it because the muscle is lengthened. In this sense, strength training perfectly complements flexibility training. Yet the myths of strength training persist. One of my goals is to dispel these myths, particularly for child athletes.

Proper strength training can reduce your child's risk of minor muscular injuries because stronger muscles are better able to resist the normal stresses of sports. In addition to strengthening soft tissues (muscles, ligaments, and tendons), training can also strengthen your child's bones and joints, thereby increasing their resistance to mechanical injury and helping to combat degenerative diseases like osteoporosis. In that sense it's true preventive medicine. A strength training program will also enhance your youngster's performance in any sport.

Methods of Developing Muscular Strength

Strength training exercises can be divided into two categories, static and dynamic. In static strength training the muscle doesn't change length. The most common static technique is isometrics. Isometric exercises are useful for maintaining muscle tone and can moderately improve muscle strength. If your child is nine years old or younger or recovering from a sports injury or surgery, then isometric exercises are ideal. They are performed by pushing against an immovable object such as a door frame, a wall, or even the nonexercising limb. Because a muscle doesn't lengthen during isometrics, it should be exercised at three or four different lengths. Each muscle contraction should last for six to ten seconds. The contractions can be repeated any number of times, but four for each joint position is sufficient.

In dynamic strength training, the muscles do change length. The three types of dynamic strength training are constant resistance, variable resistance, and accommodating resistance. Constant resistance is the most widely used method of developing strength. Both accommodating resistance (isokinetics) and variable resistance involve expensive equipment not generally available to kids, so I won't discuss them here. The equipment used in constant resistance strength training is the familiar free weights and multi-exercise machines (sometimes known as home gyms). These supply resistance that remains fixed throughout the range of motion.

There has been considerable confusion in the past concerning the differences between weight training and weightlifting, so before we go any further, let's make that clear. Weight training is a method of health fitness conditioning that uses weights. Weightlifting, on the other hand, is a sport in which the participant tries to lift the maximum weight possible. Young athletes should refrain from weightlifting until well after puberty if they want to participate in this sport.

Weight training for youngsters before adolescence, or strength training as I prefer to call it, has been a controversial subject for many years. Two main arguments have been made concerning the participation of young children in such programs. First, critics say that because children lack adult or even adolescent levels of male sex hormones, or *androgens*, training with weights can't produce gains in muscle strength or size, so there's no point in encouraging a child to go into such a program. Second, they allege that strength training for kids poses the threat of injury, especially to their growth plates. However, over the past several years some important studies have shown that children in an organized strength training program can become stronger. The first of these studies was conducted by me and Dr. Les Sewell, a colleague at Children's Hospital. I don't mind telling you that it astonished many in the medical community when we produced weekly 5 percent strength increases in boys and girls aged ten and eleven. Just as important as these unheard-of increases was that there were no injuries in our study group. The injuries that do occur during strength training are caused by using poor technique and lifting too much weight. In 1985 the National Strength and Conditioning Association told us that there had been no reports of growth-plate fractures or injuries in supervised strength training. With proper supervision strength training can be a safe, effective, and enjoyable activity for all young athletes, before and after puberty.

Strength Training Safety

Your child's strength training program can be safe and successful if a few simple rules are followed. Because your child is probably just learning to strength train, the emphasis should always be on proper technique and not on the amount he can lift. Proper technique includes:

- Total control over the weight at all times
- Correct breathing
- Correct body position
- Use of a "spotter" (you or a coach) whenever free weights are used, to help guide the weight into its proper position
- Concentration

Strength training must be taught and supervised by a qualified adult. If you don't have the training to do this — and let's face it, most parents don't — you should take a strength training course with your youngster. The YMCA is an excellent place to take such a course. I strongly recommend the book *Strength Training at the YMCA*, by Wayne L. Wescott, for your family. Other sources of qualified strength training instruction are certified physical therapists and exercise physiologists. The person supervising the exercises should give your child plenty of encouragement. This makes learning easy and the program more fun.

In 1985 the American Orthopedic Society for Sports Medicine sponsored a conference attended by delegations from the American Academy of Pediatrics, the American College of Sports Medicine, the National Athletic Trainers Association, the President's Council on Fitness and Sports, the U.S. Olympic Committee, and the Society of Pediatric Orthopedics. The participants stated in the published proceedings that strength training for prepubescents is "beneficial as well as safe." However, they discouraged competition and maximum lifting attempts at this age. I agree: *Under no circumstances should children attempt heavy weight–low repetition training.* Parents should exercise extra caution if their youngster is of very slight build or has been leading a sedentary life. Don't be fooled by size alone; a skinny, active kid is usually stronger than a larger, sedentary child.

Developing a Strength Training Program

Once again frequency, intensity, and duration are the key elements of any health fitness program, and strength training is no exception. A good rule of thumb for frequency is three workouts per week with one day of rest in between. For the youngster using school facilities, a Monday-Wednesday-Friday schedule works best. It's vital that your child understand that muscles need time to recover from a strength training session. A day without weight training is needed because the muscle-protein synthesis that produces increases in size and strength occurs during rest, not during the actual exercise. You and your child shouldn't subscribe to the misconception that if a little bit is good, a lot must be better.

Intensity, the effort needed to complete a particular exercise, is one of the most important and complex components of a strength training program. Intensity is measured by the size of

Age-Specific Recommendations for Weight Training

●

AGE	9–11	12–14	15–16	17+
Exercises for each body part	1	1	2	2
Sets	2	3	3–4	4–6
Repetitions	12–15	10–12	7–11	6–10
Maximum weight	Very light (50% 1RM)	Light (50–60% 1RM)	Moderate (50–70% 1RM)	Heavy (50–80% 1RM)

the weight and the number of repetitions performed. A muscle develops strength by adapting to greater demands, both in daily activities and by artificial methods such as training with weights. The greater the intensity, or "overload," the greater the increase in strength. This is known as the overload principle. However, using weights that are too heavy may impair strength development and cause injury. For your growing child, proper intensity is critical to achieving strength gains and no pain.

Parents frequently ask me how much weight their kids should be lifting. "He's twelve," they say, or "She's five feet tall." That doesn't help me at all! Different kids will train at different levels of intensity. The rule of thumb is that the weight should be between 50 to 80 percent of the child's maximum lift, known as "1RM." Children should be discouraged from training using their maximum lift because of the potential for injury. However they should be allowed to do this once in your presence to establish their maximum.

Children under the age of twelve should be doing repetitions of 50 percent of 1RM, while adolescents of sixteen and above can perform "reps" of between 50 and 80 percent of 1RM (see the box above). However, in all cases, when the weight is increased, the number of repetitions should be decreased. Otherwise your child's technique is likely to suffer because she will be struggling toward the end of the set, thus increasing the risk of injuring muscles and joints. The amount of weight should be increased gradually and only when your child is ready. You'll know when she's ready because she'll be able to perform the maximum number of sets and maximum repetitions comfortably.

- Nine- to eleven-year-olds should increase the weight when they can do two sets of fifteen repetitions for four consecutive workouts.
- Twelve- to fourteen-year-olds should be able to perform three sets of twelve repetitions for three consecutive workouts.
- Fifteen- to sixteen-year-olds should be able to perform three sets of twelve repetitions for three consecutive workouts.
- Sixteen-year-olds and older with at least two years of strength training can increase the weight after performing four sets of ten repetitions for two consecutive workouts.

Intensity also includes the speed at which exercises should be done. Some people recommend high-speed training because they say it most closely simulates the demands of most sports. Others contend that speed is irrelevant so long as the muscles being exercised are stressed through a complete range of motion. I support the latter view, so long as the exercise isn't performed too slowly. The "two-four" system is ideal: lifting the weight should take two seconds, and lowering it should take four seconds. There should be a momentary pause in the fully contracted position.

Duration in strength training refers to the amount of rest between sets and the total length of the session. For beginners the session shouldn't last longer than an hour. This gives children enough time for both exercising and rest periods. I generally recommend a rest period of fifteen to sixty seconds between sets, a regimen that also gives the cardiovascular system a workout.

Sport-Specific Strength Training

	NECK	SHOULDER	UPPER ARM	LOWER ARM	BACK	ABDOMEN	GROIN	HIP	QUADRICEPS	HAMSTRINGS	CALF	FOOT
Aerobics					X	X	X	X	X	X	X	X
Ballet		X			XX	X	X	X	XX	X	XX	X
Baseball	X	X	X	X	X	X	X	X	X	X	X	
Basketball		X	X		X	X	X	X	XX	X	XX	X
Bicycling					X	XX	X	X	XX	X	XX	X
Football	X	X	X	X	X	X	X	X	X	X	X	X
Golf	X	X	X	X	X		X	X				
Gymnastics	X	X	X	X	X	X	X	X	X	X	X	X
Hockey		X			X	X	X	X	X	X	X	X

Sport-Specific Strength Training

	NECK	SHOULDER	UPPER ARM	LOWER ARM	BACK	ABDOMEN	GROIN	HIP	QUADRICEPS	HAMSTRINGS	CALF	FOOT
Ice skating		X			X	X	X	X	X	X	X	X
Lacrosse		X	X	X			X	X	X	X		
Racket sports		X	X	X	X	X		X				
Soccer		X			X	X	XX	XX	X	X	X	
Track and field					X		X	X	X	X		
Volleyball		X	X	X	X	X	X	X	X	X	X	X

xx = special emphasis

The equipment your child uses to strength train must be safe and simple, must fit his body size, and must overload the muscles to be exercised. The two main types of equipment are machines and free weights. Both have advantages and disadvantages. The constrained design of good strength training machines provides an added safety feature compared to free weights. While one group of muscles is being exercised, the child is supported in a safe posture. Free weights can also be safe for the young strength trainer, but he must keep the weight stable through the whole movement. This requires additional strength and muscle coordination as well as more attention to technique. Regardless of the equipment used, supervision is crucial. If your child is training with weights at school, make sure that a qualified instructor is always on hand. At home you should always be present when your child is strength training.

Choosing which exercises to use is important. The choice should be based on the muscular requirements and injury risk areas of the sport your child is playing (see the table on pages 176–77). For the younger child who isn't intensively involved in sports, a *total* strength training program concentrating on the large muscle groups is recommended. The program should include at least one exercise for each major muscle group. For most sports, strength training in the following areas will also strengthen the smaller muscle groups in the major joints: quadriceps, hamstrings, lower back, abdominals, chest, upper back, shoulders, biceps, and triceps.

Weight Training Exercises

The following muscle-strengthening exercises should be included in a beginning or intermediate conditioning program. When performing any strength training exercise, your child should:

- Always use proper technique.
- Always perform an exercise through the full range of motion.
- Always have total control over the weight, moving it in a smooth, fluid motion.

Bent-over dumbbell rowing (*rear upper back and rear shoulder muscles*). While standing, place your left knee on a bench. Bend forward and put your left hand on the bench so your back is flat and parallel to the bench. Your right foot stays flat on the floor to the right of the bench. Hold a dumbbell in your right hand, palm forward, with your right elbow fully extended downward. Your back must stay straight, with your head and neck in line with your back. Smoothly pull the dumbbell up to chest level, keeping your right arm and elbow close to your body as you lift. Pause for one second when the dumbbell touches your chest and shoulder. Lower the dumbbell to the starting position. Inhale as the dumbbell is lowered and exhale as it is lifted. After the number of reps appropriate for your age, switch sides and perform the exercise on the left side.

Bench press (*chest, front shoulder, and triceps muscles*). Lie flat on a strength-training bench with both feet flat on the floor. Place both hands, approximately shoulder width apart, on the barbell resting in the overhead supports. Keep your back (lower back in particular) flat on the bench at all times.

Raise the barbell off the supports and slowly lower it until it gently touches your chest at approximately nipple level. Pause for one second and push the bar back to the starting position. In this position, make sure that your elbows are pointed outward and directly below the hands, with the forearms and upper arms forming a forty-five-degree angle. This gives your chest more of a workout. Inhale as the bar descends toward your chest and exhale as you push the bar up. A spotter must be present at the head of the bench to ensure proper replacement of the bar.

Behind-the-head press (*upper shoulder, rear neck, and triceps mus-*

cles). Sit on a chair or a bench with back support. Place a barbell on top of your shoulders behind your head or raise two dumbbells to shoulder level. The hands should be approximately shoulder width apart on the barbell. Look straight ahead and keep your back straight.

Take a deep breath and raise the barbell or dumbbells, exhaling as you push it above your head in a smooth, controlled manner. Pause for one second, then slowly lower the weight to the starting position while inhaling. Make sure that your back doesn't bend during this exercise. A spotter should stand behind you to help if needed and to make sure that the weight is always under control.

Seated dumbbell curls (*biceps and forearm muscles*). Sit on a bench or a chair with your knees bent, your feet flat on the floor, and your arms down by your sides, palms facing forward. Hold one dumbbell in each hand. Keep your back straight and your eyes looking forward. Exhale slowly as you lift the weight toward your chest. Pause for one second when the dumbbell reaches shoulder height, then slowly inhale while returning the dumbbell to the starting position.

Heel raises (*calf muscles*). Place a barbell across your shoulders or hold dumbbells in both hands at shoulder level. Step onto a two-by-four board with the front part of your feet so that the balls of the feet are higher than the heels. Your feet should be about twelve inches apart and the toes should point slightly outward.

Take a deep breath, then gently exhale as you rise on the balls of your feet. You should lift your heels off the floor as far as possible. Pause one second, then slowly return to the starting position with your heels back on the floor.

Reverse curls (*forearm muscles*). Stand with your feet shoulder width apart. Place your hands on a barbell or two dumbbells, grasping the weight from the top, not from underneath, at pelvis level. Bending both elbows, lift the weight to shoulder level, keeping the elbows close to the rib cage and exhaling as you lift. Slowly lower the weight to the starting position, inhaling as you lower it.

Wrist curls (front forearm muscles). Straddle the end of a bench, resting both forearms on the bench in front of you, palms upward, holding a barbell in both hands. Your wrists should be on the end of the bench, but your hands must be completely off the end. Roll the barbell to the tips of the fingers. This is the starting position. Close your fingers over the bar, letting the bar roll into the palms, then bend the wrists toward you, holding the weight. Hold this position for a count of one. Slowly lower the weight to the starting position by reversing the order of movement. Smoothly exhale when returning the weight to the starting position and inhale when flexing the finger ánd wrist joints.

Superman (back muscles). Lie flat on your stomach with arms and legs outstretched. Raise your arms and legs off the floor so your torso is supporting you. Hold this position for ten seconds to begin with. Gradually increase the time to sixty seconds.

Partial curl (abdominal muscles). Lie flat on your back with your hands clasped behind your neck and your knees bent at ninety degrees. Ideally your feet should be stabilized by resting your ankles on a bench or chair. Tuck your chin to your chest and tense the abdominal muscles as you bring your elbows up to touch your knees. Exhale as your abdominal muscles are tensed. Pause for one second as you touch your knees with your elbows. Then slowly descend to the starting position, inhaling and keeping your chin tucked to your chest.

Advanced bicycle (abdominal muscles). For athletes with strong abdominal muscles, the advanced bicycle can be used as a total abdominal strengthening exercise. Begin by lying flat on your back with both hands clasped behind your head, your knees slightly bent, and your feet on the floor. Tuck your chin to your chest and lift your shoulders off the floor. At the same time lift your feet six inches off the floor and hold them there. This is the starting and finishing position. The exercise is performed by bending your right knee and touching it with your left elbow over the navel. Pause for a second, then lower yourself to the starting position. Then bend the left knee and touch it with your right elbow. That is one repetition.

Although there's no doubt in the minds of most sports medicine experts, including myself, that strength and flexibility training for children is safe and beneficial, there has been considerable resistance to adopting such programs for several reasons. First of all, many parents think their children are already fit, cardio-vascularly and musculoskeletally. Somehow they think that "all kids are in shape." That's simply not true. The reason this misconception exists is that children traditionally have had plenty of spare time to be active and, as a result, they *were* fit. But today's sedentary lifestyle is not building heart-lung endurance or strength and flexibility.

Our bodies were designed to do the work of hunter-gatherers. However, most of us no longer need to do this kind of physical work to survive. A comprehensive strength and flexibility program makes an excellent "artificial" substitute for those activities that are no longer part of our daily lives. Just because it is artificial, that doesn't mean it is a poor substitute. A strength and flexibility program can be enjoyable and beneficial for the whole family. Indeed, it's important to remember that these exercises feel good. And they can help you look good as well, which is an important incentive for most people, both kids and adults. I urge you to begin such a program with your children as soon as possible.

9

• • • • •

Nutrition for the
Child Athlete

Diet plays a vital role in children's development. Throughout childhood, and especially just before and during the adolescent growth spurt, children have specific nutritional requirements that you as parents must recognize and fulfill. However, the modern American parent is faced with the task of making sense of the landslide of nutritional misinformation in the media. Our quick-fix society has become addicted to the search for a miracle diet that will transform us into ageless beauties with flat tummies and full heads of hair. Flip on the television and you're likely to encounter some well-coifed couple proclaiming the benefits of their "beer and popcorn" diet. Are we really so desperate that we eagerly turn charlatan nutritionists into best-selling authors with Malibu beach houses?

Of course we are! Americans recognize that this nation faces a chronic problem of obesity. Nowhere is it more pervasive than in our children. The U.S. Department of Health and Human Services acknowledges that between 25 and 30 percent of American children are overweight. Our reaction to these statistics is to search for complex solutions to this crisis. The attitude seems to be, "Hey, we put a man on the moon, let's use some of that technology to keep our kids fit." Perhaps it's a mark of our "sophistication" that we refuse to admit that our problems may have very simple explanations and solutions.

First, America's obesity problem is not a direct result of over-eating. Our calorie consumption has actually decreased since the turn of the century. But what we are consuming is very different, and this change in our eating habits has been devastating to our health. It's only quite recently that we've shifted our carbo-hydrate intake toward sugars rather than complex carbohy-drates — bread, pasta, potatoes, beans, and fresh fruit and veg-etables — which are far more nourishing than sugars. Unlike sugars, the complex carbohydrates can be stored for energy. Sugar's main contribution is to fool the body into being less hun-gry while contributing little to nutrition. And let's not forget its unique ability to rot teeth.

Not only that, but fat consumption has risen about 30 percent since 1910. Fat, although available to some degree for energy, is stored when it isn't needed. Unfortunately, we humans have not found a way to store fat as efficiently as camels, who pack it away in one convenient hump. In humans, fat looks unsightly and gets in the way, making it hard for the body to do its job. Amer-icans' declining consumption of fresh fruit, wheat flour, and po-tatoes over the past several generations has been met with a cor-responding rise in consumption of sugar, beef, poultry, corn syrup, soft drinks, and fast foods. Our children are especially vulnerable to advertising, which encourages them to indulge in unhealthy diet practices.

Paralleling this undesirable shift in eating habits has been a decline in the daily expenditure of calories. Even if your child is eating as little as 2,000 calories a day, she may be burning off less than that because she rides to and from school by bus and then sits in front of the "boob tube" for the rest of the day.

The nutritional problems of the inactive child concern me greatly, which is why, when testifying before the President's Council on Physical Fitness, I recommended sports and fitness activities as an antidote to the nutritional malaise that plagues America. Sports can tilt the equation — not to mention the scales — back to where they were, with calorie expenditure matching calorie intake.

Parents of child athletes have particular nutritional concerns, among them the problems of the obese or malnourished child, the female athlete's special considerations, and a wealth of hocus-pocus associated with athletes' diets and diet supplements.

Basic Nutritional Requirements for Young Athletes

Young athletes should learn that no miracle diets or magic potions will enable a five-foot-two kid to slam-dunk a basketball or give a twelve-year-old the strength to throw sixty-yard football passes. Contrary to popular belief (remember Rocky swigging his raw-egg milkshake?), vigorous exercise demands nothing extra except increased energy, which can be derived from the familiar four food groups, and more water.

Your child does not need extra protein, minerals, amino acids, or anything else if she is eating a balanced diet. Supplementing these nutrients is unnecessary, expensive, and potentially dangerous (for possible exceptions, see "Nutrition for the Young Female Athlete").

The essential daily nutrition for the child athlete can be achieved through:

- Two servings from the high-protein food group, such as meat, fish, chicken, turkey, or beans.
- Two servings from the dairy food group: milk, cheese, yogurt, or ice cream.

- Four servings from the grain food group: bread and cereal.
- Four servings from the fruit and vegetable group.

These twelve servings provide only 1,200 to 1,500 calories, but they provide a firm foundation for healthy sports participation by the young athlete. To this foundation can be added, within reason, second helpings and desserts. As Nathan J. Smith counsels in his book *Food for Life*, "First eat what you need, then eat what you want." Or as our parents told us, "If you don't eat your spinach, you can't have any ice cream!"

Ironically, organized sports may contribute to children's nutritional deficiency by encouraging fad diets, disrupting family meal times, and taking up so much time that regular eating habits become impossible. Child athletes often skip breakfast and lunch and make do with a couple of candy bars to get through practice or competition. They may not eat a large meal until evening, meaning that they are "running on empty" when they need the energy most — during afternoon sports practice. After a sports event youngsters are often so keyed up that they are unable to eat dinner. When their appetite returns, they head to the freezer for a pint of ice cream.

From the point of view of nutrition, these children are not fit for sports or fitness activities. A direct result of undernourishment is fatigue and, consequently, injuries. To ensure that your youngster is getting enough nourishment for sports, he should be weighed at least once a week. Any dramatic weight loss is a sign that his food consumption isn't keeping up with energy expenditure. Any child athlete who suddenly loses weight should be examined by the family's primary care physician.

Eating regular meals three or four times a day is the surest way to get the energy necessary for sports training and competition. Make sure your child has breakfast before leaving for school and encourage her to eat the school lunch. If necessary, provide a box lunch. There appears to be a direct correlation between the quality of a child's diet and the frequency of eating with the family. The youngster who is left to fix his own dinner is usually not eating well. For this reason, try to eat as a family unit as often as possible.

Nutritional Abuse

The absurd emphasis our society places on sports, and especially on winning, may drive athletes to tamper with their basic inherited physical makeup, often with dangerous consequences. Taking steroids is the most blatant form of this abuse, but almost as serious is nutritional abuse. I'm referring to the fad of "making weight," with athletes either starving themselves to qualify for a particular weight category or "bulking up" to become a more imposing physical presence. For adults these practices are ill advised, but for child athletes they can have disastrous consequences.

At this very moment, as many as a quarter million young American males may be deliberately starving themselves in order to make weight in wrestling. Undernourishment, dehydration, anorexia, and bulimia are just a few of the unnecessary occupational hazards of sports such as wrestling, gymnastics, figure skating, and ballet, in which athletes try to control their weight. In the short term, these practices may interfere with normal growth and development. In the long term they may impair basic health.

Bulking up is a practice almost exclusively of high school or junior high football players. They think that gorging on cola, french fries, and vitamin and protein supplements will guarantee them a ticket to the Super Bowl or at least a place on the first string. These young men may spend the off-season shuttling between the refrigerator and a weight machine. Without proper

nutritional counseling, the practice of bulking up is not only use-
less but dangerous. Weight that is gained without proper training is usually fat rather than muscle. Most often the dangerous
diet practices of bulking up result in obesity and its associated
problems.

Unfortunately, in many cases this nutritional abuse is condoned and even encouraged by coaches. Coaches need to be
properly educated as to the serious consequences of making
weight and bulking up. Mandatory certification would ensure
that all our youth coaches are apprised of the dangerous effects
of nutritional abuse. Until all coaches are certified, it's up to parents to be vigilant in this area.

These words of warning are not meant to dismiss the justifia-
ble desire of serious adolescent athletes to improve their athletic
ability by losing or gaining weight. Many young athletes wish to
lower their body fat content and increase their lean body mass.
Good! Safe and beneficial weight losses can be achieved by increasing energy expenditure and lowering calorie intake, thereby
decreasing body fat while maintaining or increasing muscle mass.
This should be done very gradually. A high school boy should
lose no more than two pounds a week, and a girl no more than
three. Crash diets hinder the normal growth process and lower
muscle mass.

There's also nothing wrong in principle with a young athlete
wanting to increase his weight in order to be more competitive.
Moderate increases in muscle may also help prevent injury. A
young football player can gain one to one and a half pounds a
week in muscle mass by adding a small extra meal to his daily
diet and undertaking several hourly sessions of weight training
a week. If the young athlete starts gaining body fat at the expense of lean muscle, the program should be modified.

Short-term glycogen loading, or carbo loading, as it's better
known, is the practice of manipulating diet and exercise to increase glycogen stores in the muscles. It is a common practice
among elite adult athletes and is the only safe and natural way

to maximize athletic performance through nutrition. However, it is not a wise practice for young athletes because its effect on growth is still unknown. Don't let your children try carbo loading.

Any special diet for a young athlete should be prescribed by a health professional and closely monitored by parents, the family physician, coaches, and, where relevant, school health officers.

The American Paradox: Malnutrition and Obesity

It is an unhappy paradox that in this land of plenty, both malnutrition and obesity are prevalent. Both conditions signify nutritional unfitness and may have serious consequences for the child athlete, both in the short term and in later life.

The problems of overweight in children are different than in adults. Obese child athletes are predisposed to certain injuries of the knee and hip. Furthermore, metabolic diseases such as hypertension, diabetes, and cardiovascular conditions appear to get started more easily in the obese child. These youngsters are also more likely to suffer from heat exhaustion. It won't surprise you to learn that obese child athletes may also suffer psychological problems. Unable to perform as well as their peers because of their condition, they are often cut from sports programs or drop out because of incessant ridicule. The resulting psychological blow can be devastating.

For reasons we have discussed, obesity is on the rise among American children. Two lifestyle changes are necessary if we are to curb this national trend and, indeed, to effect change in the individual obese child: a change in diet and an increase in exercise. These changes should be introduced prudently. We know that the obese child is at risk of sports injury, and being forced into a vigorous exercise program may lead to injury, which will only cut short the child's efforts to lose weight. Both swimming and cycling are excellent forms of preliminary exercise for the obese child.

As for diet, calorie-restricted diets for children can be dangerous, especially those dipping below 1,200 calories a day. Any diet that goes below that level should be closely monitored and directed by a physician. Remember that diets should not be a short-term forced restriction of calories but rather a permanent change in the pattern of eating.

Malnutrition is another serious problem in children's sports, albeit a more difficult one to solve. While obese children generally come from families that can afford to change their diet, malnourished athletes often come from poor households in which there is no choice in the type or amount of food served. Whatever their socioeconomic origin, all active, growing child athletes must be well nourished in order to participate in sports. Lack of nourishment will affect performance and, more significantly, sometimes retard the growth process. Malnourished athletes are more likely to be injured due to fatigue or to succumb to heat exhaustion.

It is a tragic situation in which America, the richest country on the planet, finds itself when millions of our children are hungry. But the political, economic, cultural, and social reasons for poverty are the subject of many other books and are beyond the realm of my expertise. What I am qualified to say is that as long as this situation persists, schools must take the major responsibility for teaching and providing proper nutrition and fitness for children.

Nutrition for the Young Female Athlete

Young women active in sports and fitness may have specific nutritional problems. Recent studies have found calcium and vitamin deficiencies in young female athletes who are training so hard that their menstrual periods have stopped. These young women have significantly lower bone mineral density and are therefore much more likely to sustain overuse injuries, especially stress fractures. Although I generally discourage dietary supplements, elite female athletes whose periods have been interrupted by strenuous exercise or the stress of competition may need calcium and vitamin supplements to prevent injuries now and osteoporosis later. But before your daughter takes any supplements, you should first determine whether her diet includes all the necessary nutrients. Too often a poor diet is the true cause of the problem. Be sure to consult your primary care physician on this matter.

The Pregame Meal

There are countless myths and fallacies about what the athlete should eat on game day. Until quite recently athletes were urged to consume an enormous steak before a game to ensure an excellent performance. The myth persists: it's not uncommon to hear a spectator say of a player performing at a high-energy level, "He must have been eating red meat before the game." It's also common for athletes to believe that sugar will improve their performance, and many will eat a candy bar to get the "sugar high." French rugby players are sometimes known to dissolve a teaspoon of sugar in a glass of sherry and quaff it just before the game!

We now know that Saturday's game is not played on Saturday's lunch or a magic elixir just before the game, but on the athlete's nutritional intake in the three days leading up to the contest. The pregame meal cannot improve performance, but it should complement the daily diet. However, the pregame meal certainly can hinder performance. That steak, for example, is a high-fat item that takes five or six hours to digest. If eaten two to three hours before the contest, as most pregame meals are, it will just lie in the child's stomach during competition. More appropriate is a meal that can be prepared easily on game day and that the child can take along to the field. Such a meal could include fruit juice, chicken sandwiches, jello, and cookies, which, because of their high-carbohydrate, low-fat content, may be eaten two and a half hours before the game. Other easily digestible high-carbohydrate, low-fat foods are cereal (eaten with low-fat milk), crackers, broth-style soups, vegetables, and yogurt, though admittedly, it is more difficult to persuade kids to eat these foods.

As for those candy bars that supposedly give the athletes "super energy," they are counterproductive. Eating sweets and sugary foods before exercise can actually hinder performance. The body produces insulin to carry sugar from the blood to the muscles. Exercise, like insulin, speeds the transport of sugar into the muscles. The combined effect of insulin and exercise may cause the child's blood sugar level to plummet and the child to become hypoglycemic and feel light-headed, shaky, and uncoordinated.

Of course, child athletes must drink plenty of water before and during exercise to avoid dehydration. It's important to stress to children that just because they're not thirsty doesn't mean their body doesn't require rehydration. Our thirst mechanism doesn't tell us soon enough when our bodies need water. Why is water so important when we exercise? First, the chemical reactions that produce energy to make our muscles work require water. Second, the water is our body's transport system for oxygen, nutrients, and body wastes, enabling us to exercise vigorously. Most important, it is water in the blood that transports the heat generated by vigorous exercise to the skin surface, where it can dissipate efficiently as sweat. It's clear that our bodies need plenty of water during exercise. This is especially true for children, who don't produce sweat as efficiently as adults and are therefore more susceptible to heat cramps, heat exhaustion, and heat stroke.

Young athletes should be encouraged by their coaches to drink a glass or two of water five to ten minutes before exercise and to drink at least one glass every twenty minutes during exercise. Coaches and organizers of all-day meets should schedule regular water breaks for the athletes. What about those commercial "sports drinks," such as Exceed and Gatorade? Are they suitable for kids? These drinks, which consist of electrolytes, carbohydrates, and flavors, help replace salts lost through sweat and help maintain blood sugar levels. Although recent evidence suggests that most athletes, including children, do not lose significant amounts of salt during exercise that lasts less than an hour, the loss of carbohydrates during such activity may deplete blood sugar. For this reason sports drinks like Exceed and Gatorade, which are 8 to 10 percent carbohydrates, help keep blood sugar levels up during vigorous activity. In addition, their palatable taste encourages young athletes to drink fluids during hot weather when they otherwise might ignore the need.

After strenuous exercise the young athlete's diet should continue to emphasize high-carbohydrate foods to replace depleted muscle sugar (glycogen), which is essential for energy. Only carbohydrates will rapidly replace the glycogen. Potatoes or pasta, for example, are better than steak for recovering from vigorous exercise.

We've seen that there is tremendous scope for nutritional abuse in youth sports. Obese high school football players and anorexic ballet dancers are signs of times when sports assume immense importance in our society. But there's a silver lining to this dark, ominous cloud. One of the most important functions of sports is to teach children an appreciation of what a healthy body can do. They'll discover that good nutrition is a prerequisite for a healthy body. Sports can provide them with the incentive to learn healthy nutritional practices and avoid drugs, cigarettes, and alcohol.

The key to all this is education. If child athletes are taught the basics of good nutrition, chances are they will follow that path for a lifetime. And they will in turn pass this knowledge on to their children. Just think — if you sit down and talk to your children today about nutrition for sports, you may be laying the foundation for the good health of generations of your descendants!

10

• • • • •

The Young Female Athlete:
Myths and Misconceptions

As the father of two intelligent, ambitious daughters, I've welcomed the increased opportunities for women in today's society. But as a sports doctor, I'm seeing many more injured girl athletes than ever before. Are they paying too high a price for equality with male athletes? The answer is no! If there is a price to be paid by the young female athlete, it's very low. The rewards, on the other hand, are enormous!

Federal and state equal rights laws have sparked an explosion in sports participation among girls. Our school systems are now required to provide equal access to sports facilities. And rightly so. The results have been dramatic. Not only are more girls taking part in traditional women's sports such as field hockey, basketball, gymnastics, tennis, and softball, but they are also making exciting inroads into male sports bastions such as soccer, ice hockey, baseball, rugby, and even football. As for the fitness boom of the last decade, who hasn't been caught in the slipstream of a young woman jogging, cycling, or speedwalking her way to an aerobics or dance class?

This phenomenon presents a number of important issues for the parents of an active daughter. When I meet the parents of a sports-mad girl, the first words out of their mouths are often, "Will she have particular types of injuries because she is a girl?" Their next question, just as predictable, is, "Will she be injured more often because she is a girl?"

"Female" Injuries?

For parents of sports-minded daughters, the answer to the first question is paradoxically reassuring: girls appear to suffer the same kinds of injuries as boys. Of course, there's no such thing as a "good" injury for a boy or a girl, but the fact that "sex-specific" injuries are a rarity puts to bed outdated and erroneous concerns about women and sports. The primary female sexual organs are better protected from serious athletic injury than the male organs. Serious sports injuries to the uterus or ovaries are extremely rare.

Breast injuries, a commonly heard concern for women's participation in contact sports, are among the rarest of all sports injuries. In fact, in my three-year study of four Boston area women's rugby clubs, not one breast injury was reported by those rough-and-tumble athletes. Still, providing breast protection is a trend in some girls' sports. Soccer leagues frequently alter the playing rules to allow girls to use their hands to protect their chests from the ball. Some women's hockey leagues have adopted special chest protectors. And over the last five years a number of support brassieres for women have been developed, although these are obviously designed to prevent discomfort and eventual sagging, not for protection.

Menstrual difficulties are another argument against girls' participation in vigorous sports training. In fact, the menstrual cycle seems to have no significant effect upon either participation or performance, and several studies show that strenuous athletic activity can actually decrease menstrual complaints. However, changes in the menstrual cycle are common in highly trained female athletes, and this may be worrisome to the child and her parents. These alterations occur most often in endurance athletes, such as distance runners, swimmers, or skiers and have also been reported in gymnasts, ice skaters, and dancers. Menstrual abnormalities appear to be the result of a combination of psychological and physiological stresses.

Recent studies suggest that oligomenorrhea (infrequent or scanty menstruation) may be related, at least in part, to low body fat. The percentage of body weight as fat seems to be the key factor in the starting and maintaining of regular periods. Several studies suggest that below some threshold of fatty tissue (allegedly 15 to 20 percent), periods will cease, a condition called amenorrhea. Incidentally, parents should be aware that the same hormonal response that is thought to trigger amenorrhea may also be responsible for anorexia in adolescent females.

But these findings shouldn't detract from the role of psychological factors in altering the menstrual cycle. Sports training and competition *can* help dissipate stress in teenagers, but it can also be a source of *heightened* stress, particularly in solo sports such as dance, gymnastics, and figure skating. And stress can bring on oligomenorrhea or amenorrhea.

Parents can take some comfort in a study conducted at West Point. In 1976, the first year women were allowed to enter the academy, a careful assessment was made of all freshmen women. After two months of rigorous training, 73 percent reported that they weren't menstruating. Three months later only 41 percent were still not having periods. After nine months the figure was down to 29 percent, and after fifteen months all but 7 percent had resumed menstruating regularly. Interestingly, after the initial phase of irregularity, approximately 55 percent of these West Point women reported a favorable change in their periods:

lighter flow, less cramping and discomfort, and shorter duration of flow.

As to whether menstrual irregularities among young female athletes have long-term negative effects, the evidence is again encouraging. No permanent impairment of reproductive or sexual function was found in a survey of 107 of the women's champions in the 1952 Olympic games. In fact, a 1972 study of former elite international female athletes revealed that these women had fewer complications during pregnancy and easier deliveries than was recorded for a group of normally active women and a less physically active group.

Although such reports are reassuring, recent studies of amenorrheic young athletes raise another concern: an apparent decrease in bone density in the legs and feet. Further, the incidence of stress fractures in the legs and feet appears to be significantly higher in amenorrheic athletes when compared to female athletes in similar sports who have normal periods. Clearly, a young female athlete who stops menstruating during training should have a medical evaluation. Treatment of this condition remains controversial at this stage, with some physicians recommending progesterone and estrogen hormones and calcium supplements.

My advice to parents is to take comfort in the available evidence but to be vigilant. In addition to a routine evaluation for menstrual abnormalities, a nutritional assessment, including a determination of the percentage of total body fat, is a priority for the girl athlete. If she shows signs of high stress or anxiety, psychological counseling or psychiatric treatment may be necessary. Simple corrective measures, including a change in training diet or resolution of the issues causing stress, may help correct the sports-related complaint and also avert other problems. There's little sound medical rationale for restricting normal young women from taking part in vigorous noncontact sports and several reasons to encourage such participation.

More Injuries?

The second question, whether girls sustain a higher rate of injury than boys, is more complex. Certainly there has been concern that females are at greater risk of injury from sports training than their male counterparts because of physiological differences between the sexes. The limited medical evidence available seems to show that girls sustain more injuries than boys in certain sports, but this higher rate is not due to physiological differences.

Young male and female athletes suffer many of the same macrotrauma injuries, including fractures, dislocations, and contusions. These injuries don't discriminate between boys and girls — they occur in the same way and are managed identically. But overuse injuries may be more common among girl athletes. The constantly repeated movements in running, jumping, or throwing a football, baseball, or javelin lead to stress fractures, knee complaints, certain kinds of tendinitis and bursitis, and the ubiquitous shin splints.

Overuse injuries, as we've seen, usually result from a combination of factors:

- An error in training, often "too much too soon"
- An anatomical malalignment of the bones and joints, sometimes from a previous injury
- An imbalance in strength or flexibility of the muscle-tendon units of the legs or arms
- Improper equipment, such as ill-fitting running shoes
- Improper surface for running, such as concrete instead of asphalt or dirt
- Interruption of menstrual periods

Young female athletes are especially susceptible to these problems for two main reasons: they often lack adequate long-term preparation for vigorous sports training, and they frequently begin sports training at the height of the growth spurt (between eleven and thirteen). At this stage bone growth creates tightness in the muscle-tendon units and in soft tissue, resulting in loss of flexibility in the joints.

This combination of inadequate preparation and imbalances of the muscles and tendons increases the chance of injury. After all, it takes years to condition the bones and soft tissues for vigorous athletic activity. Classical ballet, with its long tradition of physical training, requires three or more years of progressive training before a student is allowed to practice advanced techniques such as *en pointe*. Ballet instructors understand that bones and muscles take a long time to become stronger in response to increased physical demands.

I'm now seeing two overuse injuries in particular among my female patients. These are stress fractures in the back and in the legs, especially the knees. Both types are also seen in boys but are far more of a problem among girl athletes, especially those whose periods have stopped.

Stress fractures result from a series of microfractures that are unable to heal because of the frequency or intensity of the repetitive trauma. The normal response of bone to increased stress is ingenious: the microfractures heal over, and the bone rebuilds itself. And if this process occurs gradually and progressively, the bone can become significantly stronger. In addition, bone exposed to recurrent microtrauma may also increase in size, as happens to a pitcher's throwing arm. But stress fractures will occur if certain types of activities are constantly repeated and bones are denied the opportunity to heal. Athletes of all skill levels are subject to stress fractures; the most common cause is a sharp increase in the intensity or frequency of training.

The second condition I'm seeing more often among young female athletes is knee pain, most often in the form of chondromalacia patella, or patellofemoral pain syndrome. Sufferers complain of aching pain around the kneecap while walking or climbing stairs, stiffness in the knees after prolonged sitting, and occasionally the giving way of the knee.

Although the onset of these complaints may be associated with an error in training or a minor injury to the kneecap, evaluation of an athlete with this condition usually reveals a combination of problems, including muscle and tendon imbalance across the knee and one or more anatomical malalignments, such as patella alta (when the kneecap rides too high and bumps against the bottom of the thigh bone), knock-knees, and bowlegs.

One suggested explanation for the frequency of these complaints in female athletes is the width of the female pelvis. Combined with knock-knees, this physiological feature is said to cause the kneecaps to slip from side to side. However, I've found little evidence for this among my patients with this condition, and a survey of "growth films" of young male and female patients shows no significant biomechanical relationship between the width of the female pelvis and these problems. I'm far more concerned with such factors as the relative weakness of the quadriceps muscle and tightness of the hamstrings, which I attribute directly to young female athletes beginning vigorous athletic training at the height of the growth spurt.

Most often these knee problems respond well to a simple exercise program involving static straight-leg raises and a flexibility regimen. In addition, orthotic devices inside the shoe to alter the foot/ground relationship often help compensate for anatomical malalignments and at the same time increase impact absorption. I've found that more than 90 percent of my young female patients with knee pain respond well to the above techniques. As their level of straight-leg weight resistance increases to twelve or fifteen pounds with ten repetitions, their symptoms steadily subside.

Are Women Tough Enough?

I'm frequently asked by worried parents whether their daughters will be able to "take the punishment" meted out in vigorous sports participation. It's often been argued that girls are less able than boys to handle the physiological stresses of sports or to attain similar levels of cardiovascular or musculoskeletal fitness. "Not bad for a girl" is the phrase that sums up this attitude.

Until quite recently, it was assumed that girls simply didn't have the stamina for sustained endurance sports such as distance running, swimming, or skiing. Certain early fitness testing suggested that women were much less fit than males. But such studies often test male-oriented athletic skills and don't provide an accurate reflection of the female potential for fitness.

A symbol of the traditional attitude toward female athletic potential was the absence of distance running events for women until recently. In the 1928 Olympics, an 800-meter competition was added with only three weeks' notice. The previous maximum distance for women had been 300 meters! A number of the competitors were inadequately prepared and collapsed without finishing the race. The ensuing controversy set back women's distance running competition several decades. And yet, women now run in the Olympic marathon.

Recent studies of cardiovascular fitness and training for women have confirmed that the physiological response of athletically trained women to endurance stress is remarkably similar to that of their male counterparts — and far exceeds that of the untrained, unfit male who sits in front of the TV berating female athletes! Women routinely participate in the grueling triathlon, consisting of a two-and-a-half-mile swim, a 110-mile bicycle race, and a regulation marathon! When it comes to resisting heat illness in these events, women appear *at least* as well equipped as men, according to studies.

Recent longitudinal studies (following the same group of children for several years) have shown that boys and girls respond to endurance training in much the same way as adults. Once again there seems to be little difference between boys and girls in the ability to attain high levels of aerobic fitness in response to endurance training, laying to rest outdated concerns about the safety of endurance stress for children and, in particular, for girls.

Strength Gains

A more difficult question to answer is, "Are girls less able than boys to develop muscular strength?" This question is raised in relation to contact sports, in which it's assumed that a physically weaker athlete is at greater risk of injury.

It has been well documented that muscle bulk is associated with increased levels of the male sex hormone androgen. Indeed, weightlifters and bodybuilders frequently take androgens for their muscle-bulking properties. However, it must be stressed that there is no correlation between muscle bulk and muscle strength.

You've no doubt noticed, and many scientific studies have documented, the increase in both muscle size and strength in males at puberty. Both developments are attributed to the rising levels of androgen in boys at this age. Conversely, girls show little or no increase in strength at puberty. However, the difference in *upper* body strength between boys and girls is much more pronounced than the difference in *lower* body strength, on average. It has been frequently observed that women have less upper body strength, and this was one of the most striking results of the previously mentioned study of female West Point freshmen.

Although girls have, on average, less muscle strength than boys, when they undertake a systematic program of weight training, their strength increases are very similar to boys'. When male and female athletes of similar size and weight and, more important, of similarly lean body mass were compared, the increases of both upper *and* lower body strength after a weight training program were much the same for both sexes. The men's average *levels* of muscular strength were higher than those of the women, and this difference may indeed reflect hormonal differences between the sexes.

I can't stress enough that weight training, properly done as part of an athletic training program, not only improves the performance of female athletes but also helps decrease their injury rates by strengthening muscles, tendons, ligaments, and bones. Unfortunately, many young women in sports have stayed away from weight training for fear of becoming "hulks." Recent studies, however, reveal that weight training is not accompanied by muscle bulking in most women. Regular exercise supplemented by systematic weight training also helps establish and maintain sufficient bone mineral density, a prerequisite for avoiding osteoporosis in later life.

What remains puzzling is the difference between upper and lower body strength in boys and girls. Different androgen levels do not satisfactorily explain this anomaly; if that were the only factor, it would result in an *overall* difference in strength. I can only conclude that the main difference between male and female strength is not physiological but social. Why? Because our society still prescribes different roles for men and women after puberty. Usually a boy performs far more upper-body work and muscle training than a girl in daily life. For example, girls who are climbing trees or jungle gyms with boys at age nine will stop before the teenage years. At thirteen it's quite common for boys to lift weights while girls avoid such "macho" activities. On the other hand, there's less difference between males and females in lower-body strength after puberty. A girl may have been admonished to "behave like a lady" and give up climbing trees and wrestling with her brother in the back yard, but she doesn't stop standing, walking, or running, all of which contribute to lower-body strength.

Performance Differences

One basis for the misconception that women are much weaker than men, and therefore more prone to injury, is the difference in performance of male and female athletes. At present, top male athletes ski faster, run faster, and jump higher than their female peers. Both individual and team sports hold separate competitions based on sex, and many coaches and athletes seem determined to maintain this situation, citing the "unfairness" of mixed-sex competition or the potential for injury.

So far, however, no clear relationship has been established among strength, performance, and injury risk. And while separate competitions may be more enjoyable and comfortable for some participants, they may soon be found to be no "safer" or "fairer" than mixed competition. At the Olympics women and men compete together in one sport — equestrian events. There is no difference in injury rate between males and females in the riding events, and no claims that the men have an advantage.

Psychological Considerations

The final issue to be explored in discussing your daughter's participation in sports is the traditional concern that girls are not psychologically geared to the stresses of athletic competition. Although long-term studies are lacking, a recent study of the effect of high-level competition on the personality and adjustment of female athletes is reassuring. Elite girl swimmers who competed between 1956 and 1970 responded to a questionnaire assessing the current state of their social and familial relationships. The participants appeared to have achieved and sustained a high level of success in these relationships. They stressed that competition in no way adversely affected their development as adults in professional or male-female relationships. This certainly should put to rest fears that the physical and emotional demands of sports retard girls' social and psychological development.

God didn't create a "fairer sex" — we did. Throughout history women have been prevented from fulfilling their potential — athletic *and* otherwise — by a male-dominated society. When it came to sports, women were deemed too weak and frail to compete in demanding athletic events.

We're now discovering that if given opportunities to participate at an early age, girls run no greater risk of injury in vigorous sports than boys. According to a newly released study by the National Athletic Trainers Association, the risk of injury to female high school basketball players is identical to that of males in the almost 20,000 high schools in the United States. Of 379,000 male and 318,000 female players, 23 percent were forced to the sidelines by injury at least once during the 1987–88 season.

Parents have every reason to encourage their daughters to take part in sports and no reason to discourage their participation. By restricting their participation early on, parents may be putting their daughters at greater risk later if and when they develop an interest in sports. Finally, they will enjoy all the physical and emotional benefits of vigorous athletic endeavor.

Women have come a long way in sports, as in society as a whole. If we continue to change our attitudes for the better, they'll go a lot farther!

11

• • • • •

Sports and Recreation for the Handicapped Child

Parents of able-bodied children: don't skip this chapter. Instead, read on for a better appreciation of sports, children, and the strength of the human spirit.

I firmly believe that one of the prerequisites for a civilized society is the humane treatment of its less fortunate members. For that reason I'm extremely encouraged by the strides that have been made in care for handicapped Americans. Some may object to my enthusiasm, perhaps feeling that we have not come nearly far enough, and I will concede that there's more to be done. But this shouldn't obscure the advances we've made in providing for our handicapped brothers and sisters. Nowhere is there more evidence of our progress than in the area of sports participation for those with handicaps.

It is very important to remember that children with a disability have the same basic needs and motivational drives as able-bodied children. These needs and drives are fundamental to social growth and maturation. In addition, exercise is important for their physical development, as it is for other children. In the early years exercise is essential for the development of heart-lung endurance and the strength of bones, muscles, and ligaments.

Sports can assist in the process of physical therapy. Significantly, some physical movements that handicapped children are not able to make in a therapy program they can do routinely in sports and games. Sports inspire these kids to focus intently on what they're doing, particularly in competition with others, and not on their disability. Sports can also help control weight, build endurance, and develop strength, coordination, and control.

But sports for the disabled serve as much, much more than an extension of traditional physical therapy. If the sport is properly structured and supervised, it can help the youngster develop character, become assimilated into society, and learn coping skills. Sports may become the child's primary pleasure in life. Picture the thrill of competition in wheelchair basketball or the sheer exhilaration of water skiing for an amputee or a blind child. Outdoor leisure activities can provide a wonderful sense of freedom for the handicapped youngster. Hang gliding, horseback riding, white water rafting — imagine their appeal for those who are wheelchair-bound!

We'll see that the scope of sports participation for the handicapped child is enormous, thanks to technical advances, social changes, and medical research. But these opportunities are quite recent, so it's worthwhile to put these advances in context in order to better appreciate them.

Rehabilitative medicine is a relatively new addition to traditional medical specialties. The original pioneers were nineteenth-century Europeans, including Louis Braille, Maria Montessori, and Jean Jacques Rousseau. But over the last half century the United States has become the acknowledged leader in research, services, and programs for people with physical and mental disabilities. America's contribution has been to systematize the care of the handicapped and to bring into the field specialists in engineering, speech therapy, audiology, psychiatry, psychology, and dance therapy. What characterizes this approach is increased organization and a more inclusive plan of care — in other words, a team approach to helping handicapped individuals achieve their full potential.

In this country the most dynamic efforts to systematically assess disabilities and to improve the quality of life for the handicapped have come primarily from two very different disciplines: pediatrics and military medicine.

The campaign to help children with physical disabilities was spearheaded by Franklin Delano Roosevelt in the 1930s with the formation of the National Foundation for Infantile Paralysis. The publicity generated by his involvement led to the establishment of Crippled Children's Services in most states, providing orthopedic and medical care to handicapped children. Most of the resources of these groups were focused on corrective surgery, bracing and splinting, and physical therapy to maintain strength and function. These efforts continue to this day. However, the initial programs were quite limited in scope. The goal was to have handicapped persons be "community-ambulant," able to move about in the community under their own steam and perform daily tasks, including work and household chores.

A much more comprehensive approach to rehabilitation was inspired by federal legislation in the 1960s that made it illegal to deny handicapped people access to any federally funded sports facility. One result was the vital addition of the physical educator or coach with specific skills in sports and fitness programs for the handicapped. Programs today go far beyond physical therapy; although many of the games involve therapeutic exercises, their structure is that of a game or sport, and they require the supervision skills of a sports specialist.

The Vietnam War, with its unprecedented increase in leg injuries from land mines, ushered in a more comprehensive approach to military rehabilitation. One of the criteria for rehabilitation was participation in sports. The Veterans Administration Hospital in Boulder, Colorado, played an important role in developing riding and skiing programs for the handicapped and these programs were later expanded to include disabled civilians, including children.

Physical therapy to improve the range of motion and develop strength and coordination in the traditional hospital or outpatient physical therapy unit is often perceived by patients as laborious, painful, or boring. But when these exercises are incorporated into a sport or fitness program, they become a challenge to be mastered as well as a source of pure fun. At a recent conference on dance medicine, I was told by several colleagues about highly successful programs as diverse as dance exercise for children with cerebral palsy and dance therapy for geriatric amputees.

Much of the impetus for and innovation in sports for the disabled has come from the athletes themselves, many of whom have had no patience with the kid-glove approach that our society has demonstrated toward activities for the handicapped. Special ski equipment, lightweight pylons for canoeing or kayaking, and lightweight, low-friction wheelchairs made from thermoplastics and aluminum are just a few examples of accessories that have been developed in direct response to enthusiastic client demand. Technical advances in the design of wheelchairs, prosthetics, outrigger skis, and special weight training equipment have made sports and fitness activities even more accessible for the disabled.

What's next for sports therapy for the disabled? Two areas in which a great deal more research is needed are multiple sclerosis and muscular dystrophy.

Multiple sclerosis (MS) is a neurological disorder of unknown cause that results in a progressive loss of coordination, muscle strength, flexibility, and locomotor function. Traditionally, persons with MS have been advised to be conservative in physical therapy and to avoid vigorous activity. Many MS sufferers, frustrated with the medical establishment's cautious approach, have claimed that strenuous exercise improved both their physical and psychological well-being. Former Olympic skier Jimmy Huega, in particular, called to the attention of the National Multiple Sclerosis Foundation the need for clearer guidelines for sports and exercise for those with MS. This resulted in the publication of a manual with guidelines for systematic and symmetrical exercises, such as biking and swimming, as well as simple techniques for injury prevention.

Muscular dystrophy is another handicapping disease in which many questions remain about the appropriateness of sports and fitness activities. Therapeutic exercises are used in the care of children with muscular dystrophy, but the main emphasis has been on lifting light weights to prevent muscle contractures and maintain mobility. Although progressive weight training to overload the remaining healthy muscles seems like a logical therapy, and has been used to rehabilitate polio patients, it has never received strong support in the management of children or adults with muscular dystrophy. Yet many patients have made remarkable improvements using free weights, Nautilus equipment, or isotonic techniques. The use of these techniques for people with muscle disease deserves much more attention.

Of course, a great deal more research needs to be done in the area of sports therapy for the disabled. Initial research is very encouraging and bodes well for finding even more ways in which sports and exercise can be incorporated into rehabilitation. Coaches, physical educators, and sports physicians are now part of the handicapped care team and must continue to work with parents to encourage sports and fitness as a vital tool of rehabilitation and therapy.

Picking a Sport

Able-bodied children have different personalities, motivation, and physical abilities, and these differences are reflected in the sports they choose. The same goes for children with handicaps. They should be given the opportunity to try a number of activities so they can settle on one or several that suit their ability and temperament.

Several special conditions need to be kept in mind. First, of course, the sport should be safe and should provide the opportunity for success. Another important consideration is the nature of the disability: children recovering from illness, injury, or amputation should be encouraged to pick a sport or fitness activity that will accommodate their increasing strength and endurance. Those stricken with a relentlessly progressive disease, such as MS or cerebral palsy, should be steered toward activities that can be done regardless of their degenerating physical condition.

Needless to say, the sport shouldn't pose the threat of injury because of the youngster's particular handicap. For example, children with Down's syndrome often have an unstable upper spine, which predisposes them to serious sports injuries; children with neuromuscular disorders such as MS and muscular dystrophy may be more susceptible to heat exhaustion. The presports physical is extremely important for the disabled youngster. The physician can recommend a rate and intensity of training that will improve the child's performance and health and avoid injury.

Money is an important consideration. It's tragic that any disabled child should be denied the chance to participate in a sport or fitness activity simply because of financial considerations. But the sad fact is that some sports for the disabled require extremely expensive equipment, and the family's financial situation is often precarious enough.

The disabled child can participate in either *competitive* or *recreational* sports and fitness activities. Of course, many of the so-called competitive sports — swimming, basketball, and skiing for example — can be played for recreation. And certain recreational sports, such as golf, fishing, and sailing, can be part of a competition or tournament. But on the whole, in competitive

sports the participants are graded according to well-defined performance skills. In recreational sports, on the other hand, the
outcome of the event is secondary to the participation of all, regardless of the severity of handicap. The leisure-oriented recreational sports may be better suited to severely disabled athletes. Whatever the choice, both competitive and recreational
sports occupy a very special place in the lives of many disabled
adults and children.

Competitive Sports

Competition is often absent from traditional physical therapy
programs, but the urge to compete against others is a basic human instinct. In the case of the disabled child, arousing this instinct may help therapy and rehabilitation. As Sir Ludwig Gutt-
man, the renowned twentieth-century pioneer of sports for the
disabled, put it, "Sports puts the fight back into the fighter."

Most competitive sports for the disabled are geared toward
wheelchair-bound, lower-body-impaired adult athletes. The National Wheelchair Basketball Association was formed in 1948,
and wheelchair basketball remained the most popular sport for
the disabled. Today more than 24 regional conferences have a
total of 110 wheelchair teams that compete in a fiercely con-
tested annual national championship. The success of wheelchair
basketball paved the way for many other wheelchair sports, including archery, badminton, bowling, croquet, dance, fencing,
horseshoes, table tennis, weightlifting, and track and field. Popular team sports include basketball, softball, football, and water
polo.

For many years the medical establishment was concerned about
the effects of endurance sports on disabled athletes, but a wide

range of these sports, including the twenty-six-mile marathon, has emerged and swept away most concerns.

Modifications in rules and equipment for wheelchair sports are often necessary but are usually minor. In general, the athlete must compete from a wheelchair of a certain size and weight and must not be strapped to the chair. However, the essential character of the game remains the same. For example, in the shot-put and the discus, the chair must not cross the line of the throwing circle.

Here are some competitive sports in which modifications enable disabled athletes to participate safely and successfully.

Archery, one of the first competitive activities available to the disabled, was the sole sport featured at the first Disabled Games in England in 1948. One reason for its popularity is that it is one of the few sports in which the disabled athlete can compete at the same level as the able-bodied archer. The sole requirement is that the archer hold the grip of the bow with one hand (a stabilizer may be used), while the fingers of the other hand draw, hold, and then release the string. The drawbacks are that there aren't separate classifications based on the degree of disability and quadriplegics are unable to participate with much success.

Swimming holds an honored place in rehabilitating disabled children, so it's not surprising that it has evolved into a competitive sport. All competitive swimming events for the disabled begin in the water. Severely disabled athletes compete in twenty-five-yard events in the crawl, back stroke, and breast stroke. Those with less severe disabilities participate in longer-distance events and medleys.

Track and field has emerged as a popular opportunity for handicapped athletes, which is a tribute to their resolve, not to mention the imagination and inventiveness of the organizers. Wheelchair track competitions feature sprints of 40, 60, 100, and 220 yards, as well as the more demanding middle distances of 800 and 1,500 yards. Slalom is a particularly challenging event involving platforms, ramps, and obstacle courses. The wheel-chair marathon requires great strength and stamina. Because wheelchairs travel faster than most foot racers, especially going downhill, in many marathons they start slightly earlier to avoid collisions.

Field events for the wheelchair athlete include discus, shot-put, javelin, and precision javelin, which involves throwing at a target (the distance is 33 feet for men, 23 feet for women). The wheelchair pentathlon includes archery, swimming, javelin, shot-put, and sprint.

Fencing was introduced as an international wheelchair competitive event in the early 1970s. The three events are foil, saber, and epée. The international governing body of fencing, the Fédération Internationale d'Escrime, has made several modifications of the rules for wheelchair athletes. Most important, the wheelchair must be secured within a fencing frame so that the opposing fencers are parallel to each other and at an angle of fifteen to twenty degrees to the median line. Maximum heights for the wheelchair seat and armrests have also been established, and neither fencer is allowed to lift himself during the duel.

Unfortunately, only the lower-limb disabled can compete effectively in tournament fencing. Upper-limb-disabled athletes usually lack the balance and the essential wrist and hand functions to firmly grasp the weapon, as well as the triceps function needed to extend the elbow for the thrust. Successful fencers usually have good upper-body strength and agility.

Basketball for the wheelchair-bound was conceived in 1948 in veterans' hospitals in Massachusetts and California and has since become the most popular wheelchair sport in the United States. Its popularity is not surprising because wheelchair basketball incorporates endurance, teamwork, and precision.

Several important modifications have been made to the sport to accommodate the disabled athlete, most notably in the tip-off and the dribble. In the tip-off, players are prohibited from lifting themselves from their seats to get an advantage, as is true in most wheelchair sports. Violating this fundamental rule constitutes a "physical advantage foul" and is treated like any other foul. A player who commits three of these fouls is taken out of the game. To dribble, the player bounces the ball with one hand while wheeling the chair with the other. Or she can bounce the ball after every two pushes of the chair but must bounce the ball again before shooting or passing. In addition, play must stop when a player falls out of her chair, but only if she is obstructing play. The traditional basketball three-second zone becomes a six-second zone.

The most interesting innovation in wheelchair basketball is the way point values are assigned to players based on their disability. The International Sports for the Disabled Association has standardized guidelines to allow fair competition between participants with different degrees of handicaps. A Class I athlete is assigned one point, a Class II athlete two points, and a Class III athlete three points. At no time can the total number of points of the five players on the court add up to more than twelve. This innovation gives more severely disabled athletes the opportunity to participate.

Not surprisingly, the proliferation of sports for the disabled has led to a dramatic increase in the number of competitive events. The National Wheelchair Games, held annually since 1957, is a huge event featuring track, field, swimming, weightlifting, archery, table tennis, and the pentathlon. Other organizations that regulate wheelchair sports and sponsor national competitions include the National Wheelchair Softball Association, the National Federation of Wheelchair Tennis, the Wheelchair Bowling Association, and the Wheelchair Road Racers Club. Both horseback riding and football for the wheelchair-bound are ready to organize on a national basis.

In conjunction with the rise of wheelchair sports has been the rise of competition for ambulatory disabled athletes, who are ineligible for wheelchair events. The 1970s saw the emergence of sports meets for people with cerebral palsy, which led to the formation of the National Association of Sports for Cerebral Palsy (NASCP) in 1978. The national NASCP meet is held in odd-numbered years. An international meet is held in even-numbered years and in conjunction with the Disabled Olympics every four years. Events for athletes with cerebral palsy include archery, horseback riding, power lifting, table tennis, wheelchair and ambulant soccer, boccie, bowling, rifle shooting, and track and field.

The National Handicapped Sports and Recreation Association (NHSRA) was founded in 1972 solely for ambulatory athletes, and it attracts many amputees. This organization is especially active in teaching downhill and cross-country skiing at its headquarters in Winter Park, Colorado. The NHSRA organizes regional ski competitions, leading up to a national event each March in Winter Park.

The Special Olympics began in 1968 in Soldier Field in Chicago as a competition for people with mental and physical disabilities. Today it is the most visible of all meets because of its Olympic seal of approval and its expert organization of local and county meets. Local, area, and chapter games are held in all fifty states and the District of Columbia and in twenty-four foreign countries. Participants range in age from eight years to adults and compete in track and field, swimming, gymnastics, bowling, ice skating, basketball, and other sports. Special coaching is available for retarded children.

Recreational Sports

Like able-bodied children, many disabled athletes don't have the time or inclination for competitive sports. Also, the severity of their disability may prevent them from competing. In both cases, recreational sports may be the answer. The benefits of recreational sports, which run the gamut from scuba diving to sky diving to horseback riding, are immense. Several are useful aids to traditional physical therapy. Softball and golf provide some mild competition while emphasizing participation for all. Most recreational sports are played outdoors and provide a welcome respite for both children and parents from the tedium of indoor therapy. But above all, recreational sports are fun!

Water sports provide a range of activities for the disabled, including fly, float, and deep sea fishing, canoeing, kayaking, rowing, sculling, sailing, water skiing, power boating, snorkeling, and scuba diving. Lower-limb amputees have described fishing and swimming as among the most enjoyable recreational sports available. Scuba diving is another very popular water sport. The amputee scuba diver uses a specially shortened wet suit worn with flippers attached to the suit legs just below the stomach.

Technical advances have made fishing a highly popular and enjoyable activity for the handicapped. A harness or a fixed, vise-type pole holder allows for one-handed fishing. Special lightweight rods, spinning reels, and several other special devices for the handicapped fisherman are available by mail order from companies such as Orvis, L. L. Bean, and Abercrombie and Fitch.

Slalom water skiing, a favorite of single-leg amputees, requires strength and balance but provides speed and sheer exhilaration. Only the stand-up ski is used, and no special equipment is necessary. Water skiing is enjoyed by the blind as well as arm amputees. Even severely disabled quadriplegics can water ski thanks to the recent development of special "sleds."

Adventure sports are increasingly popular with disabled athletes. It has often been said that one of the main voids in the disabled child's life is risk. That's why disabled youngsters get such a thrill from looking down at the oh-so-distant ground from the saddle of a horse or feeling the water rush past and the wind in their hair when water skiing. Adventure sports, such as hang gliding, sky diving, parasailing behind a car or boat, and mountain climbing, have done even more to fill this void. Of course, parents should be very aware of safety considerations in these sports; if their children are interested in any of them, expert instruction is an absolute must.

Team sports for recreation should be structured for the benefit of all participants, regardless of the severity of handicap. All children want to be part of a team effort, and disabled kids are no exception. Team sports also help develop social skills, and because many disabled children have limited opportunities for social interaction with their peers, these sports should be encouraged. Popular recreational team sports include softball, soccer, football, and volleyball. Rules can be amended by the person in charge to suit the facilities and the participants. The most important consideration is safety for all the children, but this concern should be carefully balanced with the need to challenge them. Team sports can be modified in many ways to make them safe and enjoyable for disabled youngsters (see the box on pages 220–21).

Winter sports have long been enjoyed by amputees, thanks to some innovative modifications. These have led to serious competition but have also created a thriving recreational skiing subculture, which has recently been extended to those with more severe handicaps. The recent development of the Arroya sled, which is controlled by the rider shifting his weight, has opened doors for quadriplegics interested in skiing. Those with severe disabilities can be tethered to a trailing skier by a safety line. One of the pluses of recreational skiing is the extraordinary support system it offers, particularly to the newcomer or the severely handicapped athlete.

Horseback riding is now recognized as a valuable tool in treating physically and mentally handicapped children. As a form of exercise, riding improves balance, coordination, strength, posture, and rhythm. Socially, handicapped children have the opportu-

Modifications in Team Sports
for Handicapped Children

●

General

Allow children in wheelchairs or on crutches to substitute these forms of locomotion for running.

Have players walk instead of run.

Reduce the speed of the activity.

Increase the number of players on the team.

Hold the hand of a blind child when running.

Shorten the playing time.

Use a heavy balloon instead of a ball.

Put a bell in the ball for blind children.

Make the field or court smaller.

Baseball or Softball

Use a batting tee instead of a pitcher.

Pitch in an arc as in slow-pitch softball.

Have an adult pitch.

Do not have strikeouts or walks.

Shorten the pitching distance.

Provide a designated runner for the batter.

Allow the fielder to stop and kick the ball.

Basketball

Lower the baskets.

Shorten the free-shot line.

Liberalize dribbling rules.

Use wheelchairs.

Modifications in Team Sports
for Handicapped Children

●

Football

Use flag or tag instead of tackling.

Change blocking rules to disallow leaving the feet in.

Soccer

Reduce the size of the field.

Eliminate running.

Reduce the goal size.

Change the size of the ball.

Volleyball

Use a throw for the serve.

Allow catching and throwing.

Eliminate rapid movements.

Lower the net.

Increase the number of times the ball may be hit.

Allow lower-limb hits.

Let blind players have designated servers.

Adapted from B. F. LeVeau, "Team Sports," in *Recreation for the Disabled Child*, edited by Donna Bernhardt (New York: Haworth Press, 1985). Used with permission.

---

nity to meet a variety of people, including instructors, aides, parents of other riders, and other riders themselves in an atmosphere that is as different from the structured indoor world of physical therapy as one can imagine.

*

I'll leave you with a short poem written by John Anthony Davis, a British doctor who is a great admirer of riding therapy for the disabled. It deals specifically with the benefits of horseback riding, but this delightful little poem captures the essence of recreational sports for handicapped children.

> I saw a child who couldn't walk
> sit on a horse, laugh and talk
> then ride it through a field of daisies
> and yet he could not walk unaided.
> I saw a child no legs below
> Sit on a horse, and make it go.
> Through woods of green
> and places he had never been
> to sit and stare, except from a chair.
> I saw a child who could only crawl
> mount a horse and sit up tall.
> put it through degrees of paces
> and laugh at the wonder of our faces.
> I saw a child born into strife
> Take up and hold the reins of life
> And that same child, I heard him say
> Thank God for showing me the way.

12

• • • • •

Sports for the Child
with Chronic Illness

All children want to belong, to participate with their peers in free play and, increasingly, in organized sports. Until recently, children with chronic illnesses such as asthma, diabetes, and epilepsy were not allowed to take part in sports and fitness activities. With organized sports such a dominant feature of our children's lives now, those who are prevented from participating feel truly alienated. Just consider the feelings of the young asthmatic who has to endure his friends' endless descriptions of Saturday's "awesome" soccer game.

In certain respects the child with a chronic illness has a harder time than the disabled child because his condition isn't visible. Unlike a blind child or the youngster with muscular dystrophy, the asthmatic or epileptic seems normal to his friends. As a result peers often have far less sympathy and respect for these kids. Children with chronic illnesses tend to withdraw from peer activities. Even more troubling is the evidence suggesting that these youngsters are at great risk of becoming substance abusers to "prove themselves" to their peers. It is not uncommon for children who feel left out to try to earn the respect of their schoolmates by taking drugs.

One of the most exciting benefits of modern sports medicine has been advances that enable children with chronic illnesses to safely and successfully participate in strenuous sports activities. Drugs now exist that prevent the occurrence of exercise-induced symptoms and acute attacks associated with these conditions. And exercise regimens have been developed to alleviate these illnesses. It has also been determined which sports and exercise regimens are likely to precipitate an attack. These developments have progressed to the point that the American Academy of Pediatrics recently had to liberalize the American Medical Association's criteria for disqualification from sports because the previous ones were no longer relevant.

These breakthroughs are extremely important when we realize that sports and fitness are essential for children's physical and psychological development. Unfortunately, many parents are either unaware of these recent developments or are unwilling to have their chronically ill youngster take part in strenuous exercise. This is understandable. After all, one of the most difficult hurdles for any parent is a child's growing independence, which is an essential part of the transition into adulthood. If the child suffers from a disorder such as asthma, diabetes, or epilepsy, "letting go" is all the more difficult. Overprotecting and spoiling a child is a common way for parents, especially healthy parents, to work through the guilt they feel for bringing a "sickly" child into the world.

But the consequences of sheltering a child can be profound. Chronically ill children may initially strive for independence then succumb to their parents' overprotectiveness. And many kids find that it's easier to play the role of the invalid than to compete in the classroom or on the playing field. In many instances the youngster's natural drive and competitive instinct evaporate. Above all, sheltering a child from the natural hurly-burly of growing up only reinforces the feeling of being "different."

We now know that almost all children can participate in sports and fitness activities, including those with handicaps and chronic illness. Sports and fitness may be even more important for children with serious medical conditions than for those in good health. In the vast majority of cases exercise actually improves medical conditions. There is strong evidence that asthmatics, diabetics, and epileptics benefit from physical activity. And the psychological boost that sports and fitness activities give these kids is immeasurable.

I remember a young diabetic, whom I'll call Mary, who came to Children's Hospital for a pre-sports physical. Upon the advice of her primary care physician, Mary had never been allowed to participate in strenuous physical activity. Her parents won't mind my telling you that when I first saw her, Mary was shy, withdrawn, and really down on herself. After an in-depth assessment of her condition, I told Mary's parents that with careful monitoring, she could safely and successfully participate in sports. A year later I saw Mary for her next pre-sports physical. What a difference! She could hardly wait to tell me about the fun she was having playing for her high school junior varsity lacrosse team and about all the friends she had made on the team. I have seen this scenario repeated dozens of times.

The benefits of sports for children with chronic illnesses far outweigh the risks. Which is not to say that there are no risks. It is absolutely essential that before starting any sport, the child with a serious medical condition have a physical exam conducted by a physician who understands her particular condition. If your primary care physician insists that your child can't take part in sports, you should look for a physician with the knowledge and concern to explore the possibilities. Even youngsters with severe medical conditions will benefit from an appropriate sport or fitness activity, and participation is infinitely preferable to a lonely, sedentary childhood.

Asthma

Asthma is a disabling lung disorder characterized by wheezing and shortness of breath. It is such a common illness — an estimated eight million Americans suffer from asthma — that there's almost no need to describe its symptoms because surely everyone knows an asthmatic, be it a friend, relative, or colleague. Most physicians are familiar with the diagnosis and treatment of asthma, but much less is known about exercise-induced asthma. As the name suggests, this condition is brought on only by exercise. If your child shows signs of being out of breath even after mild exertion, he should be checked out for exercise-induced asthma. In our sedentary society, many people with this condition never recognize the symptoms for what they are.

Most cases of exercise-induced asthma begin in childhood. The youngster soon learns that physical exertion causes discomfort, though he may not recognize the symptoms. He may start to avoid exercise and become withdrawn, solitary, and sedentary. Because they can't exercise without suffering an asthma attack, these youngsters often think they are "unathletic." The tragedy is that they stay fixed in this pattern of behavior. In simple terms, they drop out. The primary care physician may not recognize the condition as exercise-induced asthma. Parents may attribute the child's unwillingness to participate in sports and fitness to a lack of "drive" or competitive spirit. Children with exercise-induced asthma are at high risk of becoming obese and are unlikely to develop good heart-lung and bone-muscle fitness. As adults, they become vulnerable to a host of diseases of disuse, including heart disease, lower-back pain, and osteoporosis. Not surprisingly, they often adapt to the workplace as they did to school — by avoiding strenuous activity. These children grow up believing they are suited only to desk jobs. Most don't know that they are asthmatics, and therefore they don't seek treatment to improve their condition. But with proper diagnosis and treatment, their world can expand dramatically. Asthma is one condition for which drug treatment can be truly liberating.

How can asthmatics and exercise-induced asthmatics safely and successfully participate in strenuous sports? Asthma itself is no reason to avoid exercise. The vast majority of asthmatics show no deterioration of lung function even as a result of repeated attacks. If the asthmatic takes medication to prevent attacks during exercise, her capacity to exercise should be as great as the next person's. In fact, numerous asthmatics have competed in the Olympics, most notably gold medal sprinter Jackie Joyner-Kersee at the 1988 games. The International Olympic Committee has sanctioned several drugs for competition, including terbutaline sulfate and cromolyn sodium, both of which help prevent asthma attacks. Theophyllines, the most common of which is aminophylline, are also highly effective when taken before exercise.

Yes, drugs are essential, but so is physical training, which can dramatically improve the asthmatic's ability to resist attacks. Because running for more than six minutes may trigger an asthma attack, short-duration "interval training" regimens are the most effective for improving lung function. Most exercise programs for asthmatics stress a combination of running and rest or running and walking. The intervals should be short: two minutes of running and four minutes of rest, building up to five minutes of running and ten minutes of walking or rest. Eventually, through a properly conducted exercise program, asthmatic children will be able to increase their heart-lung endurance considerably. Several coaches have told me that the asthmatics in their programs show fewer symptoms as the season progresses, but when the season is over and they get out of condition, these youngsters report a much higher incidence of asthma attacks. This fact reinforces the need for cardiovascular conditioning for asthmatics.

One of the most important decisions for the asthmatic and parents is the right sport. Outdoor endurance sports, such as soccer and cross-country skiing, are the most likely to trigger an asthma attack, particularly in a cold, dry environment. Sports that mix short bursts of activity with rest periods, such as baseball, tennis, and sprints, are more suitable. Indoor swimming, with its warmth and high humidity, is perhaps the ideal sport for the asthmatic child. A combination of conditioning, drugs, breathing exercises, and the right sport will enable the vast majority of children with lung disorders such as asthma to participate safely and successfully and to receive all the physical benefits and pure enjoyment that sports offer.

Diabetes

The situation is still unclear concerning strenuous physical activity for diabetics, particularly children. It has long been recognized that exercise benefits the diabetic by lowering blood sugar levels, but the medical profession has been slow to advocate exercise as a treatment for this condition. This cautiousness exists because the two types of diabetes — Type I, or child-onset diabetes, and Type II, often known as adult-onset diabetes — are very different.

The most common symptoms of adult-onset diabetes are excessive urination, thirst, hunger, weight loss, and weakness. Fortunately, Type II diabetes is often controllable through diet alone. For the obese diabetic, exercise is a fundamental component of treatment.

But Type I diabetes, which afflicts children, is far more difficult to treat. The symptoms include those mentioned above, along with less common, more worrisome symptoms including loss of vision, slow healing of cuts and bruises, intense skin itching (especially in the vaginal area), pain or numbness in the fingers and toes, and drowsiness. Although it hasn't yet been definitely shown that the Type I diabetic benefits from exercise, some recent, albeit controversial, evidence suggests that with proper monitoring and close attention to controlling obesity, Type I children should be able to participate fully in all types of exercise, including contact and collision sports.

Certain precautions should be taken in caring for the sports-active Type I diabetic child. If insulin is injected into a part of the body needed for vigorous movement, such as a jogger's leg, exercise may dangerously accelerate the absorption of insulin into the system. A sudden burst of insulin, especially during exercise, may cause a serious insulin reaction. For this reason it is best to inject the hormone into the abdominal wall or the fatty area of the buttock.

Most diabetic specialists who treat athletes will allow their patients to run a slightly elevated blood sugar level just before exercise. The Type I diabetic should eat before exercising and take a glucose supplement hourly during prolonged exercise.

When diabetics begin a regular exercise program, they may reduce their insulin dosage by as much as 20 to 40 percent, then test their urine four times a day to monitor their sugar level. After some experience, diabetic athletes adapt to their condition by eating more rather than by lowering their insulin dosage. A warning sign: if acidosis is indicated by the presence of ketones in the urine, then the normal control mechanisms may not be working properly and exercise may be aggravating the diabetes. In some cases ketoacidosis and diabetic coma may occur. On the other hand, if there is too much insulin in the system, energy supplies to the muscles may be impaired. Of course, no changes in dosage or schedule should be made except on the advice of a physician.

All this is to say that even Type I diabetes is not an automatic barrier to exercise. Indeed, many highly successful athletes are diabetics. But the diabetic child athlete must be cared for by a physician who is very knowledgeable about both Type I diabetic treatment and the effect of strenuous physical activity on the patient.

Epilepsy

Almost all of the available evidence suggests that exercise is beneficial for epileptics. In fact, the intense concentration that most sports demand means that he is unlikely to have a seizure during practice or play. One of the greatest benefits of participating in a sport is the feeling of self-confidence that it gives the epileptic, which further decreases the likelihood of seizures.

Nevertheless, some concerns remain about epileptics participating in vigorous sports and fitness activities. The most serious problem is the potential for harm if the epileptic does experience a seizure. Swimming is often used as an example of a sport in which an epileptic is at risk. There have been cases of drowning among epileptic children, but the risk appears to be minuscule. In a study of child drownings in Hawaii and Australia, only 4 percent of 1,000 drownings were attributed to epilepsy, and these occurred in the bathtub. The American Academy of Pediatrics has stated, "An epileptic child may swim in confidence provided he has been free of seizures for a year, has an adequate blood anticonvulsal level, and is supervised in the water by an adult."

For obvious reasons, epileptics have been discouraged from participating in many of the adventure sports, such as rock climbing, sky diving, and parasailing, in which even a minor seizure could have tragic consequences. The same is true for sports such as riflery, archery, and weight lifting. However, it is important to bear in mind that seizures are least likely to occur during these concentration-intensive activities. Seizures are most likely to happen during inactive states, especially during rest or sleep.

New therapy techniques for the treatment of epilepsy, coupled with a more complete understanding of this condition, have allowed children with controlled seizures to participate in virtually all sports. But again, the epileptic child athlete must first be seen by a knowledgeable doctor.

A Word about AIDS

AIDS is such a recent issue in children's sports that it escaped the American Academy of Pediatrics' 1986–87 review of the twelve-year-old American Medical Association guidelines for disqualification from sports. But one need only turn on the television or pick up a newspaper to understand the extent to which the specter of AIDS has influenced the way Americans think. Many of the reactions to AIDS have been overly alarmist, verging on the hysterical concerning the possibility of children being exposed to this dread disease. Not surprisingly, the issue of children with AIDS in sports is highly charged and emotional. "What if a kid with AIDS gets cut in sports and bleeds on my kid?" is not an illogical question. The chances of this happening are infinitesimal. However, until further study is done on this subject, it is probably best to err on the side of caution. The Center for Disease Control's guidelines for exposure to and handling of body secretions preclude the participation of children with AIDS in contact or collision sports. Above all, it is essential that we not succumb to the sensationalist approach that has been taken in dealing with this tragic disease.

One benefit of the prominence of sports personalities in our society has been the destigmatization of chronic illnesses through the frank admission by famous athletes of their medical conditions. What a boost it is for the chronically ill youngster to know that Olympic sprinter Jackie Joyner-Kersee is an asthmatic, or that baseball stars Don Santo and "Catfish" Hunter are diabetics. These and many other athletes have delivered to our youth the important message that chronic illness isn't an automatic barrier to athletic excellence. Of course, the vast majority of children, chronically ill or not, won't reach the same dizzying heights as these athletes. But by the same token, they shouldn't have to stay home, peering out of the window from behind the curtain while their friends and siblings are engaged in the rough-and-tumble sports and games of childhood. Instead, these youngsters should be allowed the same normal, healthy, and wholesome sports experience as other children.

13

• • • • •

Substance Abuse
and Children's Sports

How did we arrive at a time when so many of our children are dependent on alcohol or addicted to drugs — dying or being permanently damaged by substance abuse? For many of us, it's as if we woke up one morning to find terms like "crack," "smack," "freebasing," and "beer shotgunning" in the youth lexicon. But we should have seen this problem coming. For years alcohol and drugs have been tightening their grip on American children, and two generations of adults have mostly ignored this evil trend. Finally the situation is so bad that adults are forced to do something about it. The statistics paint a chilling picture:

• Alcohol-related auto accidents are the leading cause of death among teens.
• One in ten teens is dependent on drugs or alcohol.
• One in ten male adolescents has used steroids.

Perhaps we shouldn't be surprised that it has come to this. Society sends mixed messages to kids. We tell them it's wrong to abuse drugs and alcohol, yet all around them swirls a maelstrom of inducements to do just that. It's difficult for children to respect adults' scoldings about drugs and alcohol when many parents come home and enjoy three martinis before dinner every evening. If you give a cocktail party at which everybody has one too many, you may think that your kids are too young to recognize what's going on, but believe me, they're learning some very profound lessons as they peek between the stair railings at the goings-on.

We really do live in a drug culture, and I'm not talking just about illegal drugs like marijuana and cocaine. Our society's reliance on prescription drugs has created a climate in which substance abuse can flourish. Kids look at their parents taking pills to feel up, to relax, to get more fiber, or to lose weight, and they say to themselves, "Why shouldn't I smoke some pot or snort some cocaine to make me feel better?" Modern pharmacology has helped many people with genuine ailments — asthmatics and epileptics, for example — but too often, drugs are used as a shortcut to a "better" life, often with disastrous consequences. Addiction to prescription drugs is an enormous problem in the United States.

Even responsible parents are unable to shelter their children from the drug culture we live in. Hollywood is partly responsible for making drugs and alcohol glamorous, but thankfully the movie and TV industry is cleaning up its act and portraying drugs more realistically. Alcohol is a different story. Drunks are often still portrayed as happy-go-lucky, lovable characters, even when they're stumbling around knocking things over, Dudley Moore–style. The advertising industry glamorizes beer on television and hard liquor anywhere and everywhere, from magazines to freeway billboards to placards in the subway, all within plain view of our impressionable children. Most of these advertisements are selling booze to young people by portraying young, attractive models doing active things like skiing and playing touch football. The implication is clear — drinking and sports go hand in hand.

Drugs are out there, alcohol is out there. How do we stop our kids from abusing these potentially life-threatening substances?

I say abusing because I think it's unrealistic for us to expect our children not to experiment. Parents who don't believe that sometime along the way their kids are going to take a drag on a cigarette, a slug of Scotch, or a puff of a "joint" are hiding their heads in the sand — or have the luxury of living on a desert island! Children are always trying to push the limits as they approach adulthood, and peer pressure plays a major role. Kids forever egg each other on to do things they know their parents disapprove of, from listening to heavy metal bands to smoking cigarettes. Saying no to their peers is awfully hard. Our job as parents isn't to be everywhere our kids are, ready to step in and snatch the beer can or cigarette from their hands. Instead, we should help them develop defense mechanisms to resist society's negative inducements and the pressures they're exposed to.

Sports and fitness activities can be one of the most powerful of these defense mechanisms. Sports keep children busy. Kids often use drugs and alcohol because they're bored, because they feel there's nothing exciting or worthwhile in their lives. Feeling like part of a team and competing against themselves and others gives them the thrills and the sense of belonging they need. Kids who lead sedentary lives use drugs and alcohol partly because they don't realize that these substances are harming their bodies. Sports-active children know exactly how their bodies work when they're in shape, and they can feel the negative effects of drugs, alcohol, and cigarettes on their sports performance. But most important, sports give children the self-esteem they need to stand up to peer pressure. Youngsters who feel good about themselves and their bodies are much more likely to resist the cajoling of those who want them to smoke or use drugs and alcohol. It's sad that it has to be this way, but sports also give kids a valid and "honorable" excuse not to follow the crowd. "I'm an athlete," your son can say coolly to his friends when they offer him something. And in the best-case scenario his friends will not only respect this position but also emulate it.

Now here's the bad news. While sports will discourage most children from abusing drugs and alcohol, some sports situations may provide an environment in which substance abuse is either condoned or encouraged. Just as a positive sports experience can help children develop the self-esteem they need to resist negative peer pressure, a bad sports experience may do the opposite. Kids who are cut from a program or who are humiliated to the extent that they quit have suffered a severe blow. Some will turn to drugs or alcohol to feel better.

A program in which kids are pushed to the point of injury is just as bad. One young football player I treated for an overuse back injury told me, "In my school there are 'jocks,' 'brains,' and 'druggies.' I'm not a brain, and now I can't play sports. I guess there's only one thing left, isn't there?" That comment really brought home to me the powerful peer pressures at work in our children's lives: this young man needed something to boost his self-esteem, and if academics and sports weren't available to him, he was damn well going to "make it" as a drug user. Making sure our children have a safe and successful sports experience can help safeguard them against drugs and alcohol abuse. Given that many kids spend more time with the coach than they do with parents or teachers, it seems obvious to me that coaches should be drafted into the frontlines of the war against drugs, as I discuss later.

I divide substance abuse in sports into two categories, "recreational" and "performance enhancing." Both are serious problems in organized children's sports.

Recreational Substance Abuse

The so-called recreational drugs have always been part of the adult sports scene, especially if we include alcohol. But it is only

in the past quarter century or so that we have witnessed a proliferation of dangerous drugs among children. What's changed?
First, modern science has developed many more drugs, both for
good and for evil. Many of these are used by children, athletes
and nonathletes alike. But part of the allure of drugs and alcohol is their well-publicized popularity among professional athletes. The media elevate professional sportsmen and sports-
women to demigod status, then take perverse pleasure in exposing
their foibles. Just as young athletes emulate their sports heroes'
hairstyles and the way they dress, so too do they sometimes copy
their substance abuse.

The use of chewing tobacco — snuff, looseleaf, and plug, as it
is variously known — is a perfect example of this sincerest form
of flattery gone wrong. Without a doubt, many youngsters who
use chewing tobacco are copying professional baseball players
who chew it during televised games in front of millions of people. Even though they'll never be able to play baseball like their
heroes, they can chew tobacco with the best of them. What these
kids don't know is that there are numerous hazards associated
with chewing tobacco. Bad breath, cavities, and yellowing teeth
are three of the more benign consequences. More seriously, long-
term users of chewing tobacco increase by fifty times their chance
of developing oral cancer. Even moderate use quadruples the
risk. Not surprisingly, one of America's best-known baseball heroes is a glaring example of the dangers of chewing tobacco:
Babe Ruth, a heavy user of chewing tobacco, died from throat
cancer at age fifty-two. Honus Wagner, a player who was an out-
spoken critic of chewing tobacco, retired three years after Ruth
signed his first professional contract, yet he outlived Ruth by
seven years, dying in 1955 at the age of eighty-one.

Contrary to popular perception, chewing tobacco is no better
for you than cigarettes. According to the *New England Journal of
Medicine,* chewing tobacco users have the same blood nicotine
levels as smokers. And those who use two tins of chewing tobacco a week experience the same withdrawal as smokers who

go through two packs of cigarettes a day. The symptoms of withdrawal are decreased heart rate, sleep disorders, irritability, anxiety, restlessness, and difficulty concentrating.

Marijuana *is* a harmful drug, no matter what you've heard to the contrary. It is also about three times as potent as it was in the 1960s due to changes in the way it is grown. Parents who tried "pot" in their youth should be aware that the product today's kids are smoking is much more dangerous. Studies have shown chronic lung disease in those who smoke marijuana regularly. It contains more cancer-causing agents than tobacco does. And because pot smokers try to hold the smoke in their lungs for as long as possible, one joint may be as damaging to the lungs as four tobacco cigarettes. Marijuana can also affect reproductive capabilities. Women who smoke pot during pregnancy may give birth to babies with birth abnormalities, including low body weight and small heads. One marijuana cigarette affects driving skills for at least four to six hours. In combination with alcohol, marijuana can be lethal. Like alcohol, marijuana is a "gateway" drug, meaning that many youngsters who end up in drug treatment programs for cocaine or heroin addiction started with marijuana.

Alcohol has been part of the sports culture as long as sports have been around. Today the association between alcohol and sports is reinforced by the beer advertisers, who saturate televised sports events with commercials portraying active, healthy young men and women doing active, healthy things. Too often, parents give tacit approval to their kids' use of alcohol in the hope that a "harmless" taste for beer will keep them away from hard-core drugs. But parents should understand that many heavy drug users began as child abusers of alcohol and marijuana. The consequences of long-term use of alcohol are also very serious. They include high blood pressure, nerve degeneration, gastrointestinal problems, damage to the heart and other muscles, brain degeneration, confusion, severe memory problems, sleep disorders, and psychosis. Even if your child isn't a heavy regular user of alcohol, the dangers of occasional reckless drunkenness are well documented. Automobile accidents are the most frequent killers of American adolescents, and alcohol is almost always implicated in these fatalities. All too often these accidents occur on nights of great celebration — prom night or the night after the "big game."

If alcohol is one of the oldest substances abused by man, cocaine is the newest. It has become increasingly popular among athletes because along with its recreational use, it is considered a performance enhancer. Part of the problem is cocaine's availability. Until recently cocaine use was restricted to a privileged but foolish few, but now it is available on many street corners and at a much lower price. "Crack" cocaine, the culmination of this democratization, is a cheap, extremely powerful drug that is immediately addictive. It's available to anyone with a few extra dollars in their pockets, and that includes our kids. Almost one in five American teens tries cocaine. The National Institute for Drug Abuse (NIDA) reports that groups of teenagers will buy cocaine in quantity and dilute it more than adults do. NIDA's analysis of data from interviews with hotline callers aged thirteen to nineteen found that the typical caller was a white (83 percent), male (65 percent) high school junior or senior (average age 16.2 years). Many were from middle- and upper-class homes with annual incomes over $25,000. Even though cocaine is now available to many more people of differing ages and socioeconomic backgrounds, it nevertheless retains its glamour factor, especially given its apparent popularity among entertainers and athletes. Their well-publicized tales of high living too often impress young admirers, who revere these athletes to the extent that they copy their drug habits. It's a pity that kids usually see only the glamorous side of cocaine use among their sports heroes. For every celebrity who manages to play in spite of addiction, thousands are living in obscurity and poverty because of

their cocaine dependence. And even those who appear to be able
to play professional sports and abuse cocaine at the same time
find their careers cut short, along with the big money that en-
abled them to support their habit. It is well established that cocaine is highly addictive and can cause heart palpitations, seizures, and death. Some people have died after ingesting just two
"lines" of cocaine.

The signs of cocaine use by children are alternating periods
of hyperactivity and lethargy. Appetite is often suppressed. The
young cocaine user often has a persistent sniffle or postnasal
drip. A child suffering from the severe effects of cocaine may
be confused, incoherent, paranoid, and anxious and may have
headaches and heart palpitations. It's also known that cocaine
affects adolescents differently from adults. For example, adolescents have a higher rate of cocaine-related brain seizures, suicide
attempts, and violent behavior. Adolescents also find it more difficult to conceal or compensate for their cocaine addiction. The
time between first use and "deteriorating functioning" averaged
one and a half years in adolescents, compared to four years in
adults. It is *essential* that any child with a cocaine problem be
taken for drug counseling.

Performance Enhancers

As the name suggests, performance enhancers (ergogenics, as
they're properly known) include any substance that is thought
to improve an athlete's playing ability. Although performance
enhancers have come into the public eye only in the last twenty
years or so, they are not a purely modern phenomenon. Am-
sterdam's canal swimmers used stimulants as early as the 1860s.
The six-day cycle races, which originated in France in 1869, were
rife with substance abuse: the French took massive quantities of

caffeine, the Belgians ingested sugar-coated ether, and other competitors used combinations of alcohol and nitroglycerine. An English cyclist in the six-day event died of an overdose of trimethyl given to him by his manager. In the 1904 Olympics an American cyclist took strychnine sulphate. Over the next few decades the use and abuse of drugs in sports was rampant. Eventually the growing number of drug-related fatalities in sports sparked a public outcry, which eventually led to the introduction of drug testing at the 1968 Olympics. Today the use of performance enhancers has become so widespread that expensive drug testing procedures have become the norm at almost all track and field events. Those whose urine reveals traces of any prohibited substance are severely penalized.

So there's nothing new about athletes using performance enhancers. What is new is their current prevalence among young athletes. Most of those who take these drugs do so to improve their athletic prowess. The stakes in children's sports now are often so high that many kids will do anything to give themselves a competitive edge. Peer pressure soon comes into play, and certain sports programs are rife with abuse of performance-enhancing drugs. Perhaps the most insidious form of pressure occurs when a youngster who really doesn't want to use these drugs feels he has to in order to be competitive.

Needless to say, when parents and coaches turn a blind eye to the use of performance-enhancing drugs, or even encourage it, then we know we're in trouble. Too many parents and coaches get so wrapped up in the "winning is everything" attitude that if there's a drug that will help turn a child into a top performer, they'll go out of their way to get their hands on it. I've often heard the excuse that since children can get the drug anyway, it's better that they use it under a doctor's supervision. This is a thinly disguised excuse for parents and coaches to experience athletic success vicariously through the child. Perhaps if everyone — parents, coaches, and young athletes — knew more about the effects of most performance-enhancing drugs on the growth process there would be a great deal less of this abuse in children's sports.

These drugs are divided into three different groups: anabolic-androgenic agents, stimulants, and relaxants.

Steroids are the best known of the anabolic-androgenic agents and are increasingly popular among young athletes who want to improve their athletic ability or simply bulk up for appearance's sake. The use of steroids by child athletes has troubled me for years, but I was frankly astounded by a recent study from Pennsylvania State University, which showed that as many as 6.6 percent of adolescent boys have used steroids. That's half a million boys taking a life-threatening risk just so they can supposedly build muscles! The most shocking thing about the Penn State study was that a full quarter of the boys who admitted taking steroids did it not to bulk up for football, which is bad enough, but to look good. If this isn't American society's narcissism gone completely mad, I don't know what is. As we'll see, steroids are far more likely to make young men look like freaks than like the Adonises they envision as they pop those killer pills into their mouths. Steroids are extremely dangerous, especially for children.

For a long time the medical community claimed that steroids didn't "work" for young people. However, it's now clear that when adolescents use steroids in conjunction with high-intensity workouts and an appropriate diet, they do significantly increase body mass and strength. But at what cost? Steroids have a host of dangerous and highly undesirable side effects that are especially harmful to children. The problem is that many young athletes are saying, "Before you said they didn't work, but they do. Now you say they're bad for me. Why should I believe you?" We have to come clean with our kids. Yes, steroids can improve performance and build muscles, we should tell them, but they can also do serious, even lethal, damage to the human body.

Steroids are derivatives of *testosterone,* the natural male sex hormone. During normal male puberty, testosterone is responsible for accelerating growth, which includes increasing muscle bulk and decreasing fat. It is also responsible for increasing aggression and sex drive. In simple terms, when adolescents use steroids, their maturation is speeded up and they get stronger and more muscular than they would naturally, and at an earlier age. For this reason steroids are most abused in weight lifting and throwing sports and, of course, football. But steroid use by child athletes is not confined to these sports. Because steroids give kids the power to perform high-intensity workouts without getting tired, they've also become popular with endurance athletes such as swimmers, runners, and cyclists.

Ironically, the main side effect of steroids in children is stunted growth. Steroids accelerate growth, which means that the growth plates close earlier than they should. Thus the youngster who dreams of being a giant football linebacker is more likely to be undersized. Many young men who use steroids develop abnormalities in their sexual organs, including smaller testicles and a lower sperm count. In large doses, steroids cause the body to retain salt and water, which may result in "priapism," a persistent and abnormal penis erection. Some common psychological changes seen in people using steroids are increased aggression, flying into " 'roid rages," mood swings, suicidal tendencies, and an elevated sex drive. Female athletes who use steroids may suffer from "virilization" (enlargement of the clitoris and an increase in body hair) and menstrual dysfunction. For a complete list of the harmful effects of steroids, see the box on pages 244–45.

Growth hormone is another substance being used more and more by young athletes looking to improve their appearance or fit into the biggest football uniform available. Growth hormone is produced naturally by the body's *pituitary gland,* and parents often approach physicians to administer growth hormone to their kids.

Negative Side Effects of Steroids

•

Liver

Chemical hepatitis
Risk of benign and malignant liver tumors

Male reproductive system

Decreased sperm production
Testicle shrinkage
Prostate enlargement
Risk of testicle and prostate tumors

Psychological effects

Increased aggression
Mood swings, including " 'roid rages"
Sex-drive changes

Cardiovascular system

Increased blood pressure
Decreased HDL ("good" cholesterol)

Female-specific effects

Masculinization (irreversible) including clitoral enlargement,
    increased "hairiness," and deepening voice
Menstrual changes

Youth-specific effects

Premature closure of growth plates — stunted growth
Early maturation

Immune system

Inhibition of natural defense against infection

Musculoskeletal system

Weakened tendons and ligaments, increasing risk of injury

Negative Side Effects of Steroids

●

Miscellaneous effects

Acne
Alopecia (premature baldness in men)
Gynecomastia (enlarged breasts in men)

Note: Most of these effects are temporary and reversible when the drug use ceases. As with any drugs, some of the negative effects are proportional to duration, dose, and frequency while others occur regardless of these variables.

Reproduced with the permission of John A. Lombardo, M.D.

Their rationale is that since it's "natural," there won't be any side effects. Nothing could be further from the truth. What little is known about growth hormone suggests that it is extremely dangerous. True, it will probably make most children grow, but the side effects can be dramatic. The most obvious outward signs of growth hormone use are those seen in people with acromegaly, a natural disorder in which the body's pituitary gland overproduces growth hormone, often resulting in the coarsening and deformity of bones in the face, skull, hands, and feet. The wrestler "Andre the Giant" is the best-known acromegalic. These deformities also occur in abusers of growth hormone. Many of them will also develop glucose intolerance, hypertension, and heart disease. Unfortunately, new and more efficient methods of producing growth hormone are making it cheaper, and it is more frequently seen on the black market. Parents should be vigilant in educating their children not to use growth hormone.

Amino acids are becoming popular with athletes because they are thought to stimulate the release of growth hormone. It's not yet known whether amino acids will do this or whether they're harmful, but given my experience with all anabolic-androgenic agents, I strongly advise that kids stay away from these substances.

Stimulants are widely used by athletes to ward off fatigue, decrease fat levels, and increase aggressiveness, thus improving performance. The most commonly used stimulants are amphetamines, caffeine, and cocaine.

Athletes take amphetamines for speed and endurance, as well as for appetite suppression, enabling wrestlers and other weight-graded athletes to "make weight." Although it's not clear whether amphetamines actually do improve athletes' performance, and if so, to what extent, there's enough evidence to make believers of many young athletes. However, the side effects of amphetamine use include heart palpitations, hypertension, insomnia, "the shakes," and headaches. The young athlete feeling the "high" of amphetamines may fail to acknowledge signs of fatigue, and this can lead to complete collapse. In a contact sport such as football or hockey, the aggression and recklessness brought on by amphetamines pose a bodily danger to the user *and* his opponents.

Caffeine is used for many of the same reasons as amphetamines. The difference is that while amphetamines are available only by prescription, caffeine is present in significant quantities in all kinds of legally obtainable substances such as soda, coffee, tea, and chocolate. There is evidence that caffeine benefits athletes in endurance-type sports such as bicycling and cross-country skiing. Many marathoners take caffeine in large quantities before running to boost their endurance. So far caffeine hasn't been shown to improve performance in "short-burst" events such as sprints. The side effects of caffeine abuse are well known to all coffee drinkers: the shakes, hyperactivity, headaches, insomnia, atrial arrhythmias, and excessive urination. One gram of caffeine, the equivalent of ten cups of coffee, can cause muscle tension and twitching, nervousness, an inability to relax, physical agitation, rambling train of thought, rapid breathing, and rapid, irregular heartbeat. In slightly higher doses the person may begin to act delirious. As with amphetamines, the false energy that caffeine gives the athlete can cause collapse.

And there's cocaine, which I dealt with earlier in this chapter. Cocaine has been used since the time of the Incas in the form of the coca leaf for its pleasure-giving properties. But in the last decade it has become increasingly popular as a performance enhancer. There's no proof that cocaine does enhance performance, but there's plenty of evidence that it's dangerous, as evidenced by the recent deaths of several top young athletes, just a few of the hundreds of people who die every week from cocaine overdoses. Athletes who take cocaine during sports often suffer from heart palpitations, seizures, and even heart failure. They are destined for the sports scrap heap.

Relaxants, such as alcohol and "beta blockers," are most often used as performance enhancers by elite adult athletes in sports such as archery, riflery, figure skating, and ballet to relieve jitters. Child athletes rarely use these substances for this purpose, but they should nevertheless be warned against them.

Short of catching your child in the act, how do you recognize the signs of drug and alcohol abuse? In the case of performance-enhancing drugs, especially anabolic-androgenic agents, the signs are usually unmistakable (see the box on pages 244–45). Because of the serious medical consequences of using performance enhancers, any child who is found to be using them should immediately be examined by a physician knowledgeable in this area. Psychological counseling may also be necessary.

Woman's Day magazine recently published a list of useful guidelines for detecting recreational drug use.

- Your child stops going to school regularly, cuts classes, suddenly starts getting bad grades, or becomes a discipline problem.

- Your child suddenly seems uninterested in you, the family, and old friends and activities.
- Your child suddenly becomes accident prone, doesn't sleep well, or shows extreme mood swings.
- Your child makes new friends who seem to be involved in drugs and alcohol.
- Your child changes her usual behavior and starts lying to you, stealing money from you, and leaving the house without telling you where she's going.

Parents who find out that their children are using drugs are faced with one of the most difficult dilemmas in parenting. You desperately want your child to respect what you say, but you don't want to be so severe that you drive your child away from you and toward substance abuse. How do you broach the subject with your children? First of all, you should talk to your child about alcohol and drugs. Carefully explain their negative health effects, especially on sports performance. It's also important to clear up the misconceptions perpetuated about drug and alcohol use in the media. Then it's time for you to *listen*. Turn off the TV and the stereo and take the telephone off the hook. Remember: your child is much more likely to talk to you when he receives positive verbal and nonverbal signs that you're listening.

Second, try to help your child develop a healthy self-image. Low self-esteem is one of the main reasons children aren't able to say no to alcohol and drugs. Praise your child when he does positive things. If he does something you disapprove of, criticize the action, not the child.

Third, help your child develop a strong system of values. This gives kids the criteria and the courage to make decisions based on facts rather than peer pressure.

Fourth, help your child deal with peer pressure. Explain that saying no is infinitely preferable to saying yes to something that's wrong. Help your child practice saying no in specific situations.

Act out the scenario of a friend offering drugs, alcohol, or cigarettes. Rehearse the reasons your child will give his friends for why he isn't going to follow the crowd.

Fifth, make family policies that help your child say no. The strongest support your child can have in refusing to use drugs and alcohol is the solid bonds created within the family unit. Always chaperone your children's parties. It helps if parents let other family members and friends know that drug use and the use of alcohol by minors are violations of family rules. Tell your kids that their use of drugs and alcohol is completely unacceptable within the family and spell out clearly the consequences and punishment for violations.

Sixth, encourage your child to join an antidrug club. With over 10,000 such clubs nationwide, chances are there's one in your community. If not, contact a local school principal about starting such a club. If your child plays sports, you should contact the coach about getting the whole team to join. These clubs develop positive peer pressure, strengthen children's ability to turn down drugs and alcohol, and teach kids about their harmful effects.

Finally, encourage your children to participate in healthy, creative activities that keep them away from drugs and alcohol. Sports and fitness activities are certainly one of the most effective ways of helping your child avoid drugs and alcohol. If your child's life is full, there's neither the time nor the place for drugs and alcohol. Meet the parents of your child's friends and classmates and encourage drug- and alcohol-free alternative activities. Discuss guidelines and problem areas and agree to keep in touch. Consider forming a parents' group. There's strength in numbers! Making these contacts before a problem arises may prevent the problem from developing. When your child's entire peer group is on the right track, they all stand a much better chance of remaining drug- and alcohol-free.

But what happens if drug or alcohol abuse is directly related to your child's sports participation? Then you must act quickly and decisively. Let's say you discover that your son and several of his football teammates are sneaking off after practice to drink or smoke pot. Don't immediately yank him from the program — that will only turn him against you. Instead, tell the coach what's going on. If he already knows what they're up to, then you and the other parents should inform his superiors and get a cast-iron assurance from them that the coach will work on eradicating the abuse immediately — with your help. If the coach is as much in the dark as you are, as is probably the case, you should work together to stamp out the problem.

Coaches have an especially crucial role in combating drug abuse in young athletes. They have control over their athletes for a significant amount of time, and they usually command respect from their young charges. For these reasons the Drug Enforcement Administration and the National High School Athletic Coaches Association have launched a vigorous effort to enlist the support of coaches in the fight against drug abuse.* According to DEA administrator John Lawn, "If coaches take the lead in coordinating an alcohol and drug prevention program in their athletic programs, I believe, as a former coach, that they'll be effective simply because 'coach' is behind it."

Your child's coach can take the following steps to counteract drug and alcohol abuse by the athletes:

• Call the captains together and talk about alcohol and other drug abuse.
• Open a dialogue with the athletes about drugs and alcohol.
• Get the athletes to use peer pressure on teammates to refrain from taking alcohol and drugs.
• Enforce all training rules and school regulations pertaining to drugs and alcohol.

*For free information for coaches on how to start a drug prevention program, contact: DEA, Demand Reduction Section, 1405 I St. N.W., Washington, D.C. 20537.

- Advise athletes of the legal penalties associated with using or selling drugs or alcohol.
- Learn to recognize the symptoms of abuse.
- Have a definite plan for dealing with drug and alcohol use by the athletes.
- Schedule a conference with parents for cosigning training-rule pledge cards.
- Check on athletes, call them at home, let them know their coach cares.
- Investigate any violations and confront the athlete immediately.
- Take immediate action after overhearing party plans involving alcohol or drugs.
- Confront the athlete immediately if you smell alcohol or any form of tobacco.
- Develop alternative activities for athletes.
- Set a good example for the athletes.

One of the most intriguing ideas I've heard for combating drug and alcohol abuse came to me first from Dr. Larry Friedman of Deaconess Hospital in Boston, which is right across the street from Children's Hospital. Dr. Friedman, in addition to working in youth drug rehabilitation at the hospital, runs a private drug counseling center. From his experience he tells me that it's very difficult for adults to successfully counsel children against drug and alcohol abuse; peer counseling is much more effective. Dr. Friedman suggests recruiting team captains and natural leaders to the cause. By focusing our efforts on youngsters who are held in high esteem by their peers, it's possible to create an environment in which abstaining from drugs is "cool." The DEA and the National High School Coaches Association also recommend this tactic. They suggest that captains hold a team talk and tell their teammates what they want in the area of drug and alcohol abuse, including the following:

- No one uses drugs or alcohol.
- Everyone follows the rules, even the star of the team.
- If the captain hears of alcohol or drug abuse, or sees it, he should confront the athlete and warn him once.
- The captain should do everything to stop the athlete using drugs or alcohol, including going to the coach.

It's important that the captains themselves be above reproach since they are role models for their teammates, as well as for many other young people in the community. Team captains should find activities for themselves and their teammates that don't include going to parties where alcohol or drugs are used. Such activities might include going out for pizza or to a movie or a private party at home where the host can show classic sports videotapes or a good movie, or even going camping. The team's booster club should be asked to help organize and sponsor such activities. Finally, team captains should be made aware that their job doesn't end when the final whistle of the final game of the season blows — it is a year-round responsibility!

The problem of performance-enhancing drugs can be handled in a similar manner, though coaches must play an even greater role in wiping out this scourge. Most recreational drugs are taken away from the sports environment and therefore away from the coaches' jursidiction, but performance enhancers are inextricably linked to the sports environment. Coaches need to be taught to spot the signs of performance-enhancing drug abuse, which will happen when certification of coaches becomes mandatory.

Above all, the potentially devastating physical damage wreaked by these substances must be brought to our kids' attention. If shock tactics work, I'm all in favor of them. Just the other day I received in the mail two posters devised by the advertising agency Fallon McElligott and the University of Michigan to portray the side effects of steroids. One of them shows a man with breasts and a woman with male genitals. I'd like to see those posters on the locker room walls of every high school in America, no matter how many squeamish adults they offend. I've heard of a drug counselor who begins his addresses to high school athletes this way: "Guys, if you want your balls to shrink, take steroids." Shocking? Yes. Effective? I think so.

Finally, parents must be role models. It has been well established that children of drug and alcohol abusers emulate their parents' behavior. Parents who abuse drugs and alcohol have no right to condemn their children for doing the same. It's up to you to set an example your kids can follow.

14

• • • • •

Where Do We Go
from Here?

Children's sports have undergone a revolution in the past
quarter century. In the past we could rely on informal sports
and free play to provide our kids with fun and fitness. Organized sports don't seem to be doing as good a job as their less
structured predecessors in these two areas. If they were, children wouldn't be dropping out of sports at the staggering rate
we're seeing — an estimated 70 to 80 percent quit or are cut
from the program or are severely injured before the age of fifteen. Nor would kids be getting fatter and fatter.

But organized sports do have the potential to do everything
we want them to. I see the products of excellent sports programs
every day in the form of happy, healthy, well-adjusted youngsters. However, I also see the results of poorly run, misdirected
programs: athletes with injuries or emotional problems or who
are just fed up with sports. We adults must make sure our children have as safe and successful a sports experience as possible.
But how do we do this?

We all agree that children's sports programs should be fun.
All our serious talk of character development and personal growth
boils down to this simple concept. If children are enjoying their
sports experience, the other pieces will fall into place. But if the

coach is a bad sport and a bully; if the parents show up at the games to scream "Kill 'em, Johnny!"; if the kids are forced to stand around listening to a know-it-all coach lecture on "proper technique"; if they are made to run, jump, and throw until their arms and legs *hurt*, then I'll wager your children aren't having fun.

Setting the stage for a lifetime of health fitness is another important goal of youth sports. But until very recently, coaches and parents would point out a kid and say, "Look how fast he can run; he must be fit," or, "Look how far she can hit the ball; she must be in great shape." But as we now know, sports fitness is very different from health fitness. Sports fitness is largely congenitally determined and contributes nothing to lifelong good health. Health fitness, on the other hand, can be achieved by all and can be pursued throughout life. That's why it's vital that we encourage, practice, and preach good health fitness habits at home and make sure that sports coaches do the same. We must also insist that schools and communities spend less money on elite team sports like football and hockey and much more on school and community health fitness facilities such as swimming pools, bike trails, and walking/jogging tracks. And of course, we must push for qualified coaches to make youth sports programs an environment where fun and fitness are top priorities.

I strongly believe that the root cause of most of the problems in children's sports is the preoccupation with competition. Adults stepped in, took over children's sports, and asked, "How do we make this fun?" Without thinking about what the kids wanted, adults came up with the answer: "Competitions, tournaments, leagues, trophies!" But they imposed a very adult concept on children. Yes, children love to compete, but I don't think they're that interested in competitions. When they seem to be relishing the thrill of a tournament, it's usually in response to the adults' behavior. Too often parents and coaches think "success" is quantified by the win-loss record or the team's standing in a league.

This "winning is everything" attitude detracts from the sports experience for kids.

Safety is also jeopardized by the pressure to win. In order to build a winning team, untrained coaches often put their athletes through endless, mind-numbing, intensive drills. These drills are the best way to precipitate an overuse injury, and most coaches aren't trained to recognize such injuries. When a youngster is hurting but hasn't suffered a dramatic acute injury such as a sprain or fracture, she is often accused of being a malingerer and the condition is ignored. In the name of victory, these kids continue to be pushed so hard that long-term injury is almost assured.

Just as important, children find these drills plain boring. They want to run and play the game, and that's what they should be doing to build health fitness. But instead they're made to endlessly practice their batting swing or basketball layup. Many kids quit sports altogether because they find these drills insufferable. We need trained coaches for whom winning isn't the only criterion for success, who can incorporate learning basic skills into health fitness regimens that are fun. Parents must also change their approach. The first question out of your mouth shouldn't be "Did you win?" It should be "Did you have fun?"

Another disturbing outcome of America's preoccupation with competition in youth sports is elitism. Most sports programs for late adolescents are geared to the best athletes, who represent only a tiny percentage of our kids. Along the way most children who want to participate, even those as young as nine, are told, "Look, you're just not good enough." From a very early age our kids are told not to bother with sports unless they're the biggest, the fastest, the strongest, the most coordinated. The attitude is, "Only the best need apply." We tell them they can show up to watch the games, and that's what they'll do throughout life. Yes, we're a sports-mad society — from the confines of a couch.

I'm all in favor of the United States emulating the European model of youth sports. Most European countries have a national sports and fitness policy, and coaching certification is mandatory. Most significant, competition in their programs isn't stressed until much later. It is a much more inclusive approach, not one that is preoccupied with making champions out of eight-year-olds and weeding out preteens who want to participate but who "aren't good enough." European children stay involved in sports for a much longer time and are much more likely to stay active as adults. One reason that this philosophy has been adopted in Europe is that leaders there recognize that fitness is an inexpensive, highly effective form of preventive medicine. It's in the interest of European governments to keep their citizens healthy because the state pays for medical care. Our leaders don't feel Americans' rising levels of degenerative diseases pinching at their budgets yet. But when they do feel it — and who knows how bad the situation will have to get before that happens — they will surely turn to fitness for all rather than competition for an elite few as the antidote. To achieve this goal it will be necessary to decrease competition and promote sports and health fitness for all American children.

We must dramatically reduce the emphasis on competitions, especially for our younger children. Not competitive sports, mind you, just those meaningless tournaments that teach children that it's not taking part that counts, but the shiny trophy that comes with winning. If ever there was an emblem of the inappropriateness of tournaments for young children, it lies in an image that sticks with me of a young lad who walked up to the podium to collect the enormous trophy for a Boston Under-Twelve soccer program. The trophy was almost as tall as he was! He couldn't pick it up, and he burst into tears. I've attended enough high school sports to know who really pushes these leagues, trophies, and tournaments: the adults.

Let me drive a final nail into the coffin of the argument that children need competitions to cope with life and build character.

While I was writing this book, I visited friends whose son was enrolled in a baseball program they really thought was tops. I stopped in to watch, and I couldn't have agreed more. The kids in the program, red-faced and huffing and puffing, were always on the move, always having fun. When I asked my friend's son who was winning, he said his team was. But when he dashed back into the fray, I asked the same question of a little girl on the opposing team. She thought her team was in the lead! Intrigued, I asked around and got completely different replies from these ten-year-olds. They were all doing their absolute darndest to hit the ball and make it to the next base, but they couldn't tell me which team was winning, let alone what the score was. More to the point, they didn't seem to care. However, they all had the same answer when I asked them the all-important question:

"Are you having fun?"

"Yes!"

Appendix

• • • • •

Sports, Fitness, and Health Resources

A number of national organizations provide information and services regarding sports and fitness and prevention of sports injuries. The organizations here are subdivided into Health, Safety, and Fitness; Medicine; and Sports. Following the list of organizations are descriptions of some useful sports- and fitness-related booklets and audiovisual resources.

Organizations

Health, Fitness, and Safety

American Alliance for Health, Physical Education, Recreation and Dance (AAHPERD)
1900 Association Drive
Reston, VA 22091
(703) 476-3400
Publications: *Research Quarterly, Health Education; Journal of Physical Education, Recreation and Dance.* Pamphlets include "Physical Education and Sport for the Secondary Student," "Guidelines for Children's Sports," and "Nutrition for Sports Success."

Purpose: To support, encourage, and assist member groups and their personnel in developing and conducting programs in health, leisure, and movement-related activities.

American Association for Leisure and Recreation (AALR)
1900 Association Drive
Reston, VA 22091
(703) 476-3490
Purpose: To promote school, community, and national programs of leisure services and recreation education. Affiliated with AAHPERD.

American Athletic Trainers Association (AATA) and Certification Board, Inc.
660 W. Duarte Road
Arcadia, CA 91006
(818) 445-1978
Publication: *AATA Newsletter*
Purpose: To establish national minimum competency standards for the prevention and care of athletic injuries by athletic trainers.

American Coaching Effectiveness Program
Box 5076
Champaign, IL 61820
(217) 351-5076
Purpose: To provide an educational program to increase coaches' understanding of sports medicine and science, and to help them teach sports more effectively.

American Council for Drug Education
204 Monroe Street
Rockville, MD 20850
(301) 294-0600
Purpose: To produce educational materials, review scientific findings, and develop educational media campaigns. The coun-

cil produces and distributes materials on the prevention of drug abuse in several high-risk groups, including adolescents, young working adults, women of childbearing age, and the elderly.

American National Standards Institute
1430 Broadway
New York, NY 10018
(212) 642-4900
Purpose: To coordinate development of voluntary national safety standards in sports.

American School Health Association (ASHA)
National Office
Box 708
Kent, OH 44204-0708
(216) 678-7848
Publication: *Journal of School Health*
Coordinator of Study Committees: Larry K. Olsen, Ph.D., FASHA
PEBE 208, Department of HPE
Arizona State University
Tempe, AZ 85287
(602) 965-0911
The ASHA has a number of separate study committees:
ASHA Study Committee on College Health Education and Professional Preparation
Barbara A. Rienzo, Ph.D., chairperson
Department of Health Education
Building 4, Florida Gym
University of Florida
Gainesville, FL 32611
(904) 392-0583

ASHA Study Committee on Drug Education
Susan R. Levy, Ph.D., chairperson
University of Illinois at Chicago Circle

Box 4348
Chicago, IL 60680
(312) 996-7000

ASHA Study Committee on Nutrition
Beatrice P. Largay, chairperson
7711 Livingstone Road
Oxon Hill, MD 20745
(301) 567-9616

ASHA Study Committee on Physical Activities
James W. Lochner, Ed.D., chairperson
Weber State College
Box 2801
Ogden, UT 84408
(801) 626-6140

ASHA Study Committee on Safety and Emergency Care
Ken Peden, Ed.D., FASHA, chairperson
College of Education
Clemson University
Clemson, SC 29634-0709
(803) 656-3311

ASHA Study Committee on School Health Education
Lorraine H. Jones, R.N., M.A., M.S.N., chairperson
School of Nursing
Ball State University
Muncie, IN 47306
(317) 289-1241

ASHA Study Committee on School Nurses
Alicia A. Snyder, R.N., M.A., chairperson
37 Rock Ridge Drive N.E.
Albuquerque, NM 87122
(505) 296-5146

ASHA Study Committee on School Physicians
Vivian K. Harlin, M.D., FASHA, chairperson
Box 340
Ravensdale, WA 98501
Phone national office

American Society for Testing and Materials (ASTM)
1916 Race Street
Philadelphia, PA 19103
(215) 299-5475
Publication: *ASTM 1987 Publications Catalog*
Purpose: To publish technical information to promote the understanding of technology and to ensure product safety.

American Swimming Coaches' Association
One Hall of Fame Drive
Ft. Lauderdale, FL 33316
(305) 462-6267
Publications: *A.S.C.A. Magazine, A.S.C.A. Newsletter, Journal of Research*
Purpose: To provide professional education and five levels of certification for coaches in all phases of American swimming.

Association for Research, Administration and Professional Councils and Societies (ARAPCS)
1900 Association Drive
Reston, VA 22091
(703) 476-3490
Purpose: To coordinate the activities of the following special-interest groups: aquatics, college and university administrators, city and county directors, outdoor education, physical fitness, measurement and evaluation, facilities, equipment and supplies, international relations, student members, and adapted physical activities. Affiliated with AAHPERD.

Association for the Advancement of Health Education (AAHE)

1900 Association Drive
Reston, VA 22091
(703) 476-3490
Purpose: To represent the interests of professional health educators working in schools, the community, and clinical settings. Affiliated with AAHPERD.

Athletic Information Center

Johnson & Johnson Consumer Products, Inc.
199 Grandview Road
Skillman, NJ 08558
(800) 526-3967
Publications: *Athletic Uses of Adhesive Tape,* taping guide, taping films.
Purpose: To serve consumers by providing information on all products marketed by Johnson & Johnson Consumer Products, as well as related health care information.

Center for Sports Law & Risk Management, Inc.

8080 N. Central Expressway
Suite 400
Dallas, TX 75206
(214) 360-9691
Publication: *Risk Review Manual*
Purpose: To assist school districts through a risk review program to diminish the potential for sports injuries and lawsuits, upgrade safety for sports participants and spectators, and reduce insurance costs.

Center for the Study of Sport in Society, National University Consortium for Sport in Society

Northeastern University
271 Huntington Avenue

Suite 244
Boston, MA 02115
(617) 437-5815
Publications: *Journal of Sport and Social Issues, Arena Review, CSSS News Summary*
Purpose: To instill in young athletes via school outreach programs the importance of academic standards and achievement.

Childhood Accident Injury Prevention Program
Utah Department of Health
288 North 1460 West
Box 6650
Salt Lake City, UT 84116-0650
(801) 538-6140
Purpose: To collect data on sports-related injuries occurring at school among children and adolescents.

Drug Enforcement Administration (DEA)
Public Affairs Staff
1405 I Street N.W.
Washington, DC 20537
(202) 633-1000
Publications: *For Coaches Only: How to Start a Drug Prevention Program.* A videocassette, *Say No to Drugs: It's Your Decision,* is available from Bill Butler at the above address.
Purpose: To educate the public about drug abuse. The DEA will also help arrange school talks by sports figures as part of the drug awareness program.

Exer-Safety Association
2044 Euclid Avenue
Cleveland, OH 44115
(216) 687-1718
Publication: *Exercise Safety News*

Purpose: To provide the latest information on injury prevention (particularly in exercising to music) through basic training and continuing education programs.

Fitness Motivation Institute of America
36 Harold Avenue
San Jose, CA 95117
(408) 246-9191
Publication: *FitFax*
Purpose: To improve the fitness level of all Americans.

Institute for Aerobics Research (IAR)
12330 Preston Road
Dallas, TX 75230
(214) 701-8001
Publication: *The Aerobics News*
Purpose: To promote understanding of the relationship between living habits and health to enhance the physical and emotional well-being of individuals.

**Joint Commission on Competitive Safeguards
and Medical Aspects of Sports**
Oklahoma State University Hospital and Clinic
Stillwater, OK 74078
(405) 744-7031
Purpose: To promote communication among the organizations interested in the health and safety of those engaged in athletics; to establish guidelines and research in athletic medicine; and to formulate recommendations for the rules and administration of athletic programs.

Kansas Injury Prevention Program
Kansas Department of Health and Environment
Landon State Office Building, 10th Floor
900 S.W. Jackson
Topeka, KS 66612-1290

Purpose: To prevent athletic injuries to school-age children and youth.

National Association of Governors' Councils on Physical Fitness and Sports (NAGCPFS)
Pan American Plaza
201 S. Capitol Avenue
Suite 440
Indianapolis, IN 46225
(317) 237-5630
Publication: *NAGCPFS Newsletter*

National Association of Speed and Explosion (NASE)
Box 35111
Richmond, VA 23235
(804) 794-6034
Publication: *Sportspeed*
Purpose: To disseminate information on the improvement of explosive speed and power that can be applied by coaches and athletes in all sports.

National Athletic Health Institute
575 East Hardy Street
Inglewood, CA 90301
(213) 674-1600
Purpose: To conduct research, public and professional education, and community service programs in sports medicine, cardiovascular fitness, and recreational health.

National Athletic Trainers' Association, Inc. (NATA)
1001 East Fourth Street
Greenville, NC 27858
(919) 752-1725
Publication: *Athletic Training Journal*

Purpose: To encourage and improve the athletic training profession, and to promote a better working relationship among persons interested in the problems of training.

National Dance Association
1900 Association Drive
Reston, VA 22091
(703) 476-3490
Purpose: To promote the development of sound policies for dance education through conferences, conventions, special projects, publications, and cooperation with other dance and performing arts programs. Affiliated with AAHPERD.

National High School Athletic Coaches Association
1515 East Silver Springs Boulevard
Suite 240W
Ocala, FL 32670
(904) 622-3660
Publication: *National Coach*
Purpose: To promote cooperation among coaches, administrators, press, and public. The association is becoming increasingly active in sports medicine.

National High School Athletic Trainers Committee
John Hersey High School
1900 East Thomas Avenue
Arlington Heights, IL 60004
(312) 259-8508
Purpose: To promote the profession of athletic training, teach awareness of the problems of the certified athletic trainer at the secondary school level, improve the quality of health care at the secondary school level, and improve the relationships between the National Athletic Trainers Association and the State/National High School Athletic Association.

National Institute for Fitness and Sport
901 West New York Street
Indianapolis, IN 46223
(317) 274-3432
Purpose: To promote the active lifestyle; to conduct research in exercise physiology, sports medicine, health, and fitness; and to provide services such as fitness evaluations, nutrition counseling, weight management, and stress management.

National Operating Committee on Standards for Athletic Equipment (NOCSAI)
c/o Glen Meredith, Ph.D.
11724 Plaza Circle
Box 20626
Kansas City, MO 64195
(816) 464-5470
Publication: *NOCSAE Manual*
Purpose: To commission research and establish standards for athletic equipment.

National Safety Council
Public Safety Department
444 North Michigan Avenue
Chicago, IL 60611
(312) 527-4800
Publication: *Accident Facts*
Purpose: To serve as a national resource and to produce annual national estimates of injury statistics.

National Strength and Conditioning Association (NSCA)
300 Old City Hall Landmark
916 O Street
Box 81410
Lincoln, NE 68501
(402) 472-3000

Publications: *National Strength and Conditioning Association Journal, Journal of Applied Sport Science Research*
Purpose: To facilitate the professional exchange of ideas about strength and conditioning to improve athletic performance and fitness.

National Youth Foundation
2250 East Imperial Highway
Suite 412
El Segundo, CA 90245
(213) 640-0145
Purpose: To conduct programs that encourage participation in physical fitness and sports activities. To support educational programs and to assist nonprofit tax-exempt organizations, government agencies, and public bodies that promote physical fitness.

National Youth Sports Coaches' Association
2611 Old Okeechobee Road
West Palm Beach, FL 33409
(305) 684-1141
Publications: *Insights, Youth Sports, Youth Sport Guide Book* series, cassettes, and pamphlets.
Purpose: To improve youth league sport programming; to research athletic injuries and ways to prevent them; to research communities', clubs', and institutions' requirements in education and experience for prospective coaches; to create and distribute a national Bill of Rights for Athletes; to promote awareness among parents and youth of coaching requirements; and to improve the standards for education and requirements necessary to coach sports.

National Youth Sports Foundation for
the Prevention of Athletic Injuries, Inc.
10 Meredith Circle

Needham, MA 02192
(617) 449-2499
Purpose: To ensure the well-being and safety of all youth participating in sports. It is an educational and research foundation as well as a clearinghouse for information.

North American Youth Sport Institute
4985 Oak Garden Drive
Kernersville, NC 27284
(919) 784-4926
Publications: *Sport Scene, NAYSI Resource List*
Purpose: To write, edit, research, conduct trainings, and consult in sports, recreation, education, fitness, and health for national youth organizations.

President's Council on Physical Fitness and Sports (PCPFS)
450 Fifth Street N.W.
Suite 7103
Washington, DC 20001
(202) 272-3421
Publications: *PCPFS Newsletter,* publications on fitness and physical fitness, and sports medicine bibliographic references.
Purpose: To promote physical fitness and sports participation among Americans of all ages.

Recreational Safety Institute
1500 Lakeland Avenue
Bohemia, NY 11716
(516) 563-4806
Publication: *Leisure Litigation Digest*
Purpose: To provide information and assistance and to conduct research on accident prevention and litigation.

Safety Society
1900 Association Drive

Reston, VA 22091
(703) 476-3430
Publication: *Safety Forum Newsletter*
Purpose: To prevent injury through the development and support of school and community safety programs. The society is part of the Association for Research Administration, Professional Councils and Societies (ARAPCS) of the American Alliance for Health, Physical Education, Recreation and Dance (AAHPERD).

U.S. Consumer Product Safety Commission
Office of Information and Public Affairs
Washington, DC 20207
(301) 492-6980
Publications: Numerous publications and fact sheets on product-related injuries.
Purpose: To reduce unreasonable risks of injury associated with consumer products used in homes, schools, and public places.

U.S. Gymnastics Safety Association
Box 465
Vienna, VA 22180
(703) 476-6660
Publication: *Gymnastic Safety Manual*
Purpose: To raise the level of safety in gymnastics and to provide certification for coaches.

Medicine

Academy for Sports Dentistry (ASD)
c/o Jim Gallman, D.D.S. (secretary/treasurer)
12200 Preston Road
Dallas, TX 75230
(214) 239-7223

Publication: *Sports Dentistry Newsletter*
Purpose: To promote research pertaining to sports dentistry and to communicate advancements to members.

American Academy of Orthopaedic Surgeons (AAOS)
222 S. Prospect
Park Ridge, IL 60068
(312) 823-7186
Publications: *AAOS Report, The Bulletin*
Purpose: To provide education and practice-management services for orthopedic surgeons and allied health professionals; to advocate improved patient care; and to inform the public about orthopedics. The academy has a number of committees that focus on sports-related injuries and issues.

American Academy of Pediatrics (AAP)
Committee on Sports Medicine
141 Northwest Point Boulevard
Box 927
Elk Grove Village, IL 60009-0927
(800) 433-9016 (outside of Illinois)
(800) 421-0589 (in Illinois)
Publications: A manual, checklist, and policy statement on health care for young athletes.
Purpose: To educate pediatricians and the public on exercise and fitness for children and on the care of the young athlete.

American Academy of Physical Medicine and
Rehabilitation (AAPMR)
Special Interest Group on Sports Medicine
122 S. Michigan Avenue
Suite 1300
Chicago, IL 60603
(312) 922-9366

Publications: *Archives of Physical Medicine and Rehabilitation, Journal of Physical Medicine*
Purpose: To promote interest in sports medicine and provide educational opportunities for physical medicine specialists involved in treating sports-related injuries.

American Academy of Podiatric Sports Medicine (AAPSM)
1729 Glastonberry Road
Potomac, MD 20854
(301) 424-7440
Publication: *AAPSM Newsletter*
Purpose: To promote podiatric sports medicine through education, research, and communication.

American Academy of Sports Physicians
7535 Laurel Canyon Boulevard
North Hollywood, CA 91605
(213) 877-9475
Purpose: To educate and inform physicians whose practices are mainly in sports medicine and to register and recognize physicians who have an expertise in this field.

American College of Emergency Physicians
Box 619911
Dallas, TX 75261
(214) 550-0911
Purpose: To improve the training of emergency-care physicians and the treatment available in emergency medicine departments. Makes available information on emergency medicine.

American College of Sports Medicine
P.O. Box 1440
Indianapolis, IN 46206-1440
(317) 637-9200
Publications: *Medicine and Science in Sports and Exercise, Sports Medicine Bulletin, Exercise and Sport Sciences Reviews*

Purpose: To tell members and the public about research on the effect of sports, exercise, and other activities on the health of people of all ages.

American Medical Soccer Association (AMSA)
c/o Gordon Spink, M.D.
3910 Sandlewood Drive
Okemos, MI 48864
(517) 353-4730
Publication: *AMSA Newsletter*
Purpose: To exchange medical and general information about soccer.

American Optometric Association (AOA)
Sports Vision Section (SVS)
243 N. Lindbergh Boulevard
St. Louis, MO 63141
(314) 991-4100
Publication: *SVS News and Views*
Purpose: To provide education and research in sports vision and vision evaluation and enhancement programs.

American Orthopaedic Society for Sports Medicine (AOSSM)
70 West Hubbard Street
Suite 202
Chicago, IL 60610
(312) 644-2623
Publication: *American Journal of Sports Medicine*
Purpose: To conduct educational and research programs that benefit all professionals involved in sports medicine as well as the general public.

American Osteopathic Academy of Sports Medicine
1551 N.W. 54th Street
Suite 200

Seattle, WA 98107

(206) 782-3383

Purpose: To promote education, high ethical standards, communication, and research in sports medicine.

American Physical Therapy Association (APTA)

1111 N. Fairfax Street

Alexandria, VA 22314

(703) 684-2782

Publication: *Physical Therapy*

Purpose: To promote the professional practice of, research by, and education of APTA members.

College of Health and Human Performance

University of Florida

Gainesville, FL 32611

(904) 392-0584

Publications: *ISSP Newsletter, International Journal of Sport Psychology, The Sport Psychologist*

Purpose: To promote the exchange of ideas by individuals and groups from different countries and continents, and to produce a body of scholarly knowledge in sport psychology.

Gatorade Sports Science Institute

The Quaker Oats Company

Box 81740

Chicago, IL 60681-0740

Purpose: To provide current information on developments in exercise science and sports medicine and to support the advancement of sports science research. The institute is made up of academicians and practitioners who serve on either the Education Advisory Board or the Sports Medicine Review Board.

International Federation of Sports Medicine

5800 Jeff Place

Edina, MN 55436
(612) 835-3222
Purpose: To maintain and improve physical and mental health through sporting activities.

Lake Placid Sports Medicine Society
Box 327
Lake Placid, NY 12946
(518) 523-1530
Publication: *Sports Medicine Update*
Purpose: To disseminate clinical information on the treatment of injuries in winter sports.

National Academy of Sports Vision
200 S. Prospect Avenue
Harrisburg, PA 17109
(717) 652-8080
Publication: *Sports Vision Highlights*
Purpose: To advance research and education in sports vision and to serve as a meeting place for professionals in this field.

National Collegiate Athletic Association (NCAA)
Committee on Competitive Safeguards and
Medical Aspects of Sports
Box 1906
Mission, KS 66201
(913) 384-3220
Publications: *The Sports Medicine Handbook, Injury Surveillance Annual Report*
Purpose: To optimize the conditions of student athletic competition.

Physical Medicine Research Foundation
207 West Hasting Street
Suite 215

Vancouver, BC V6B 1H7
(604) 684-4148
Publication: *Physical Medicine Newsletter*
Purpose: To pursue and fund clinical research and education in physical medicine.

Society for Adolescent Medicine
Box 3462
Granada Hills, CA 01344
Publication: *Journal of Adolescent Health Care*
Purpose: To improve the quality of adolescent health care through communication among and training of adolescent health care professionals.

Sports

Amateur Athletic Union of the United States (AAU)
AAU House
Box 68207
Indianapolis, IN 46268
(317) 872-2900
Publication: *InfoAAU*
Purpose: To improve and promote amateur sports.

Amateur Basketball Association of the United States (ABAUSA)
1750 E. Boulder Street
Colorado Springs, CO 80909
(303) 632-7687
Purpose: To serve as the national governing body for basketball. They will provide information on their programs.

Amateur Hockey Association of the United States
2997 Bradmore Valley Road

Colorado Springs, CO 80906
(719) 576-4990
Purpose: To develop and promote hockey.

Amateur Softball Association of America
2801 N.E. 50th Street
Oklahoma City, OK 73111
(405) 424-5266
Purpose: To develop and promote organized softball.

American Amateur Racquetball Association (AARA)
815 N. Weber Street
Colorado Springs, CO 80903
(303) 635-5396
Purpose: To promote racquetball. They will provide information about the sport.

American Junior Golf Association
2415 Steeplechase Lane
Roswell, GA 30076
(404) 998-4653
Publication: *AJGA Tour Talk Newsletter*
Purpose: To provide information on junior golf, rules, recruiting, and related matters.

American Legion Baseball Board
Box 105
Indianapolis, IN 46206
(317) 635-8411
Purpose: To set standards and make rules and recommendations regarding high school baseball.

Athletic Congress/U.S.A.
Box 120
Indianapolis, IN 46206
(317) 638-9155

Publications: *American Athletics Annual,* U.S. Athletics Calendar
Purpose: To serve as the national governing body for track and field, road racing, and race walking.

Athletic Institute

200 Castlewood Drive
North Palm Beach, FL 33408
(305) 842-3600
Purpose: To promote sports to the youth of America and the world by funding or providing major development assistance to amateur sports associations and by producing sports and physical education programs.

Coalition of Americans to Protect Sports (CAPS)

200 Castlewood Drive
North Palm Beach, FL 33408
(800) 338-8678
Publication: *Sports Liability News*
Purpose: To lobby for tort reform to combat liability insurance premiums and to serve as the legislative arm for the entire sports and recreation community.

International Amateur Swimming Federation (IASF)

200 Financial Center
Des Moines, IA 50309
(515) 224-1116
Purpose: To promote amateur swimming, diving, water polo, and synchronized swimming.

National Association for Girls and Women in Sports (NAGWS)

1900 Association Drive
Reston, VA 22091
(703) 476-3490
Purpose: To serve those involved in teaching, coaching, officiating, training, and administering all sports as well as club sports

and intramurals at the elementary, secondary, and college levels. The overall goal is to foster quality and equality in sports for women. Affiliated with AAHPERD.

National Association for Sport and Physical Education (NASPE)

1900 Association Drive
Reston, VA 22091
(703) 476-3490

Publications: *Journal of Physical Education and Recreation*, texts, manuals, AV aids, and books, including *Youth Sports Guide for Coaches and Parents*.

Purpose: To improve sports and physical education and to provide research and education programs, public information, conferences, and symposia. Affiliated with AAHPERD.

National Federation of Interscholastic Coaches Association

11724 Plaza Circle
Kansas City, MO 64195
(816) 464-5400

Purpose: To promote among member state associations the belief that interscholastic activities programs are essential to the education of most youth and are an integral part of school curricula.

National Intramural-Recreational Sports Association (NIRSA)

Room 221, Gill Coliseum
Oregon State University
Corvallis, OR 97331
(503) 754-2088

Publications: *NIRSA Journal, NIRSA Newsletter*

Purpose: To establish quality recreational sports programs and services.

Special Olympics
1701 K Street N.W.
Suite 203
Washington, DC 20006
(202) 331-1346
Purpose: To promote physical fitness, sports training, and athletic competition for mentally retarded children and adults. Their information packet includes a general introduction to the Special Olympics and a list of state and U.S. territory chapters.

United States Figure Skating Association
20 First Street
Colorado Springs, CO 80906
(303) 635-5200
Purpose: To serve as the governing body for amateur figure skating in the United States. Information will be provided by mail on local clubs and on learning to skate.

United States Olympic Committee
Division of Sports Medicine and Science
1750 East Boulder Street
Colorado Springs, CO 80909-5760
(719) 632-5551/578-4575
Publications: *Sports Mediscope,* brochures, pamphlets, and videotapes
Purpose: To provide services to United States amateur athletes participating in National Sports Governing Body (NGB) programs and competitions at the Olympic Training Centers and elsewhere.

United States Olympic Training Center
Sports Medicine
1776 Older Avenue
Colorado Springs, CO 80909-7760

Purpose: To promote a program of physical fitness, sports training, and athletic competition for United States amateur athletes.

United States Soccer Federation
350 Fifth Avenue, Room 4010
New York, NY 10118
(212) 736-0915
Purpose: To serve as the national governing body for soccer and as a clearinghouse for information, publications, and audiovisuals on soccer.

United States Sports Academy
One Academy Drive
Daphne, AL 36526-9552
(205) 626-3303
Purpose: To educate and certify professionals in sports via graduate education, Certified Educational Units (CEUs), and certification throughout the world.

United States Swimming, Inc.
1750 East Boulder Street
Colorado Springs, CO 80909
(303) 578-4578
Purpose: To serve as the national governing body for amateur competition swimming. They offer a variety of programs geared to all levels of swimmers.

United States Volleyball Association
1750 East Boulder Street
Colorado Springs, CO 80909
(303) 632-5551, ext. 3331
Purpose: To serve as the national governing body for volleyball. They will refer inquirers to an appropriate regional director.

Women's Sports Foundation (WSF)
342 Madison Avenue

Suite 728
New York, NY 10173
(800) 227-3988 (outside of New York)
(212) 972-9170 (in New York)
Publications: *Women's Sports and Fitness, Headway*
Purpose: To produce women's sports and serve as an information network.

Youth Sports Institute
I.M. Sports Circle Building
Michigan State University
East Lansing, MI 48824
(517) 353-6689
Publications: *Spotlight on Youth Sports Newsletter,* numerous documents on coaching, sports skills, and conditioning.
Purpose: To determine the beneficial and detrimental effects of participation in youth sports through on-campus and field-based research programs; to provide educational materials and programs for parents, coaches, officials, and admnistrators.

Booklets on Sports, Safety, and Health

The American Academy of Orthopaedic Surgeons publishes a number of useful brochures. *Cast Care* includes information on why casts are used, what they are made of, how they are applied, and how to become accustomed to and maintain them, as well as a list of warning signs that a physician should be consulted. *Fractures* explains what bones are made of and how they occur, and describes the types of fractures, their treatment, and the use of different types of casts. It includes guidelines for exercise and diet as well as tips on how to avoid fractures. A series of nine brochures describes common orthopedic problems in simple terms; the topics are: *Total Joint Replacement; Health Care Options;*

Arthritis; Low Back Pain; Sprains and Strains; Orthopedics; Common Foot Problems; Scoliosis; and *Osteoporosis.* Single copies of all of these brochures are available free of charge. Send a self-addressed, stamped, business-size envelope with the name of the brochure to American Academy of Orthopaedic Surgeons, 222 South Prospect Avenue, Park Ridge, IL 60068.

The Amateur Hockey Association of the United States publishes brochures for coaches and other officials. *A Guide for Administering a Hockey Tournament* covers all aspects of hosting a successful tournament within the association's guidelines, including a checklist of things to do. *A Guide to the Treatment of Hockey Injuries* explains how to determine and handle the injuries that occur most often in youth hockey. The Hockey Equipment Certification Council works closely with the AHAUS in developing standards for hockey equipment. The *H.E.C.C. Brochure* describes how standards are set and how equipment is certified. *The Relationship Between Coach and Parent* provides ways for coaches to deal with parents of hockey players and have them become part of the game. *Development Seminars* describes the national development programs that are available to AHAUS-registered officials, including regional, advanced, and select officials' camps; seminar instructor training sessions; regional development seminars, and preseason local seminars. To receive any of these brochures, write to the AHAUS, 2997 Broadmoor Valley Road, Colorado Springs, CO 80906. Or phone (303) 576-4990.

Nutrition and Hydration in Swimming: How They Can Affect Your Performance discusses proper nutrition and hydration for swimmers during training and competition. It tells how to develop lean rather than fat body weight and how to maintain weight through a balanced diet. The booklet, written in clear, simple language, is intended for swimmers, parents, and coaches. Send a stamped, self-addressed, business-size envelope to Ross Laboratories, 625 Cleveland Avenue, Columbus, OH 43216.

Preventing Sports Injuries in Young Children discusses preparticipation assessment, conditioning, supervision, protective equipment, warning signals, and injury guidelines. For a free single copy, send a stamped, self-addressed, business-size envelope to the Pennsylvania Easter Seal Society, 1500 Fulling Mill Road, P.O. Box 497, Middletown, PA 17507-0497.

The American College of Sports Medicine publishes lay summaries of its opinion statements on issues such as fitness, steroids, prevention of heat injuries, and other topics. To obtain a full listing, contact the ACSM at P.O. Box 1440, Indianapolis, IN 46206-1440. (317) 637-9200.

Audiovisual Resources

The American Junior Golf Association sells a promotional film for $11. Contact Bobbie DeLisle, AJGA, 2415 Steeplechase Lane, Roswell, GA 30076. (404) 998-4653.

Functional Planning: Implementing Safety and Emergency Procedures; Informed Consent; Student Injuries: The Instructor's Responsibilities and Legal Liability; Student Wellness: Drugs, Diet, and Determination; and more than fifty chemical health videotapes are available for use at no charge. They vary in length from eleven minutes to one hour. Contact Denise Collomb, Massachusetts Interscholastic Athletic Association, 83 Cedar Street, Milford, MA 01757. (508) 478-5641.

Johnson & Johnson has a series of four tapes on athletic care: *Ankle Injuries; Shoulder Injuries; Foot Injuries;* and *Knee Injuries,* $14.95 each, $59.80 the set. *Athletic Taping,* $14.95, is free if the four-tape series is ordered. They also have a series of four tapes on the pro football training room: *Shoulder and Knee Injuries; Hand, Wrist, and Elbow Injuries; Soft Tissue Injuries;* and *Neck, Head, and Facial Injuries,* $14.95 each, $59.80 the set. Contact Johnson & Johnson, 1-800-526-3967.

The Injury Factor, a documentary for parents and professionals regarding health care for secondary school athletes, is available on half-inch and three-quarter-inch VHS videocassettes. Contact the National Athletic Trainers Association, Membership Department, 1001 East Fourth Street, Greenville, NC 27858.

Sports Sense for Grades 7–12 covers the importance of proper exercise as well as prevention and treatment of sports injuries. Videotape, $15. Contact Advil Forum on Health Education, 1775 Broadway, 22nd Floor, New York, NY 10019. (212) 757-9100.

The American Hockey Association of the United States provides *I'd Rather Play Hockey* (free, 16 mm only); and a three-part series on training and conditioning for hockey: *Training for Leg Power and Quickness; Strength Training for Hockey;* and *Principles of Conditioning for Youth Hockey.* Films, $200 each; VHS tapes, $49.95 each. Contact AHAUS, 2997 Broadmoor Valley Road, Colorado Springs, CO 80906. (303) 576-4990.

Teaching films for basketball and football and rules films for baseball, basketball, football, soccer, swimming and diving, track and field, volleyball, and wrestling are available from the National Federation of State High School Associations, 11724 Plaza Circle, P.O. Box 20626, Kansas City, MO 64195.

The American Coaching Effectiveness Program has a Level 1 video package, which includes *Coaching Philosophy; Sports Psychology; Sports Pedagogy; Sports Physiology; Sports Medicine;* and *Sports Management.* Half-inch VHS tapes, $60 each; six-tape set, $300. Contact ACEP, Box 5076, Champaign, IL 61820.

A number of videotapes and slide sets with audiocassettes are available from the Health Sciences Center for Educational Resources, including: *Coach, the Athlete, and Nutrition; Common Overuse Injuries of the Lower Extremities; Common Soft Tissue Injuries; Conducting a Safe Practice; Fatness Reduction and Weight-Control Program for the High School Wrestler;* and *Today's Young Woman in Sports* ($150 each); and *First Step: Handling the Life-Threatening Emergency; Fueling the Body for Sport; The New Woman Athlete; Overuse*

Injuries: Too Much, Too Fast, Too Soon; Pathway to a Winning Season; and *Sports Injuries Today* ($85 each). Contact Distribution Coordinator, HSCER, T-281, SB-56, University of Washington, Seattle, WA 98195. (206) 545-1186.

More than one hundred audiotapes on swimming are available for $7 each, including shipping, from the American Swimming Coaches Association, One Hall of Fame Drive, Fort Lauderdale, FL 33316.

Fitness in 6 to 15 Minutes a Day the ISOROBIC Way, $49.95, can be ordered from Mary Moyer, Fitness Motivation Institute of America, 36 Harold Avenue, San Jose, CA 95117. (408) 246-9191.

Playsafe is a documentary for schools on the pre-sports physical exam. Contact Jan Stegelman, Project Coordinator, Prevention of Athletic Injuries to School-Age Children and Youth Project, Kansas Department of Health and Environment, Landon State Office Building, 10th Floor, 900 S.W. Jackson, Topeka, KS 66612-1290. (913) 296-1205.

Index

About the Authors

Dr. Lyle J. Micheli is Director of Sports Medicine at Children's Hospital, Boston, and an associate clinical professor of orthopedic surgery at the Harvard Medical School. He is a fellow of the American Academy of Orthopaedic Surgeons, the American Academy of Pediatrics, and the American College of Sports Medicine. He co-founded the world's first children's sports medicine clinic at Children's Hospital in 1974. An internationally recognized authority on sports medicine, Dr. Micheli is a keen athlete himself, having represented Harvard in football, boxing, lacrosse, and rugby in the 1950s and 1960s. When his hectic schedule permits, Dr. Micheli still occasionally pulls on his cleats for a game of "veterans' rugby." Dr. Micheli will serve as President of the American College of Sports Medicine until May 1990.

Mark D. Jenkins has covered sports and fitness for several national publications, including *Sports Illustrated,* the *Wall Street Journal, American Heritage,* and *SportCare & Fitness.*